HCG DIET
800 CALORIE
PROTOCOL
SECOND EDITION

PHYSICIAN RECOMMENDED AND APPROVED

Authored By: Sonia E. Russell, LPN

Licensed Nurse and Professional hCG Diet Coach

Foreword by Dean Yannello

Published by eBookIt.com

ISBN-13: 978-1-4566-1023-4

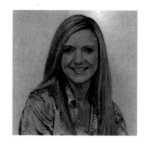

Biography of
Sonia E. Russell, LPN

I am a nurse with over 14 years of clinical experience and was trained at UCLA Medical Center in California. As a professional hCG diet coach, I have researched and tested the 800 calorie protocol on thousands of patients in the clinical setting over the past 5 years. I co-developed the modified 800 calorie protocol with a team of physicians. Our intention was to provide the dieter with a safer, more comfortable plan. We believed adding breakfast, along with additional protein and vegetables options, could produce the same, if not better, weight loss results when compared to the original 500 calorie VLCD. The protocol also includes many improvements to the original phase 3 stabilization plan by the removal of certain foods that many dieters have been known to overindulge upon.

In 2007, my medical team and I began our internal testing and food trial studies on the 800 calorie plan with our patients in the clinical setting. Additionally, in 2010 a 6-week successful clinical study was performed by the American Society of Bariatric Physicians ASBP on the modified 800 plan. http://www.weightshop.net/documents/Bryman%20HCG%20Article.pdf

In May 2011, I published our findings in my book developed specifically for the hCG dieter entitled, *HCG Diet 800 Calorie Protocol*. The 800 calorie protocol has indeed been proven safer, more comfortable, and in most cases yielded higher losses when compared to the original 500 VLCD.

I am also a co-author of the book entitled, *The Best Diet You Have Never Heard Of - Physician Updated 800 Calorie hCG Diet Removes Health Concerns.* This book was written by medical professionals for the prescribing practitioner to utilize as a higher standard for Rx hCG weight loss therapy prescribed off label for weight loss.

In 2011, I teamed up with personal fitness trainer, Candice Ekberg, B.S. ESS, NSCA-CPT, AEMT to create an expanded guide that will ensure the dieter a successful stabilization in phase 3 entitled, *Phase 3 HCG Diet: Successful Stabilization Plan Revealed.* Our purpose was to eliminate the need for chronic correction days, unnecessary additional rounds and help teach dieters how to keep the weight off for good. To learn more about how Candice lost weight utilizing the HCG Diet 800 Calorie Protocol, visit her blog at http://www.bodybycandice.com To download a copy of our phase 3 guide to your e-Reader device such as Kindle, Nook, iPad, please visit https://www.ebookit.com/books/0000001364/Phase-3-HCG-Diet-Successful-Stabilization-Plan-Revealed.html?sonia

Facebook Support Groups
HCG Diet 800 Calorie Protocol Support –
http://www.facebook.com/groups/168886913206892/
HCG Diet 800 Calorie Protocol – business page
http://www.facebook.com/groups/100738906691037/
Inches and Pounds – business page
http://www.facebook.com/inchesandpounds
Sonia E Russell – page
http://www.facebook.com/inchesadmin

To view my hCG Diet Books Library visit
http://www.hcgdoctorsgroup.com

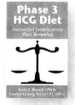 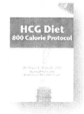 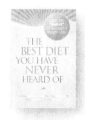 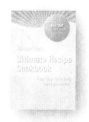

Contents

HCG Diet Facts

Recently in the news and on many popular morning talk shows, the hCG diet has been stirring up quite a bit of debate as to its safety. A large majority of medical professionals who practice traditional weight loss avoid treating their weight management patients with hCG therapy because they feel it is unsafe at 500 calories per day. There are very few doctors nationally who prescribe the hormone to their patients.

Many dieters have claimed to be weak, tired, and complain of hunger and frequent headaches on 500 calories, but have plenty of energy on the 800 without the hunger or headaches. Many report they have lost hair on 500 calories, but not on the 800 calorie plan. Dieters have also reported they have been able to lose the same if not better on the 800 and have maintained their weight loss. Those who have chosen the 800 Calorie Protocol feel it is a safer, more healthful plan. Many physicians agree and have begun incorporating the hCG diet 800 Calorie Protocol in their weight management practices.

There is so much more to the protocol revision than just adding 300 calories. These additional calories are mostly from protein sources.. Breakfast is included in the program in addition to specific nutritional supplements, more allowable foods to choose from, and more often. The 800 Calorie Protocol does not allow any canned or processed foods, fat free/sugar free store bought foods or products that contain antibiotics, preservatives, flavor enhancers, pesticides, sugar substitutes, corn syrups, herbicides, or hormones.

The obesity epidemic in America is outrageous and it is not the only country dealing with this issue. My belief is that the HCG Diet 800 Calorie Protocol will help more Americans, and hCG dieters across the globe, to lose weight safely and assist in reducing weight related disease. Positive reports on the benefits of this protocol have already come in from hCG dieters in Canada, Ireland, and the UK.

This protocol will teach the dieter how to change their past eating habits by learning the healthiest ways to grocery shop, read food labels, prepare and cook healthier foods.

Foreword

By Dean Yannello

In 2007, I owned a medical weight loss clinic and hired Sonia to work with our medical director that prescribed Rx hCG for weight loss. Little did I know that down the road she would be recognized as one of the leading experts in hCG diet therapy and weight loss safety. Today, she is now my business partner and together we have developed one of the largest coaching support groups on Facebook and have published 5 books on the 800 calorie hCG diet. I've met very few people with Sonia's passion and dedication to help others succeed in their weight loss journey. It's no surprise that her extensive research and knowledge have made her a valued resource for many physicians who wish to offer hCG as a weight loss therapy to their patients and are seeking leading-edge guidance on this protocol. Sonia has helped thousands of dieters improve their health and prevent obesity related disease. She is a shining star!

Introduction

The hCG Diet: What is it?

The hCG diet was discovered by a British endocrinologist, Dr. A.T.W. Simeons, who was always looking for cures for current-day medical problems.

Dr. Simeons had already pioneered an anti-malaria drug and studied bubonic plague and leprosy in India when he turned his attention to weight-loss and obesity in the 1950's.

One day, a woman came to his office in Rome for a weight-loss consultation. He was on the phone as she sat down and when he looked up at her, he noticed she was emaciated. Her skin was dry and loose, her collarbone and ribs protruding. He hung up the phone and was about to tell her she had the wrong doctor when she stood up. "I know you think I'm mad, but just wait."

As she rounded his desk, he saw that she had enormous hips and thighs below her small waist.

Dr. Simeons had studied a hormone called hCG (Human Chorionic Gonadotropin). hCG is-produced in the placenta of pregnant women. It converts stored body fat into nutrition for the baby.

The HCG hormone was being extracted from the urine of pregnant women and given to young boys suffering from Froehlich Syndrome. These were the so called "fat boys" with oversized breasts and undersized sexual organs. He had noticed that the HCG helped the boys lose their appetites and inches around their hips.

Dr. Simeons treated the woman with 125 IU's (international units) of pharmaceutical HCG via daily IM injections. Within 8 weeks, she lost 8 inches around her hips. He claimed by using the hCG, combined with a calorie-restricted diet and a 30 minute daily walk, the woman was able to get rid of her reserve fat.

By 1967, weight-loss patients from around the world flocked to Dr. Simeon's clinic in Rome. He was treating Hollywood starlets, royalty, the rich and famous.

He was spending enormous amounts of time telling other doctors and hospitals about his HCG diet, so he put together a protocol titled, *Pounds and Inches: A New Approach to Obesity.*

His claim: Men and women who used the hCG diet had no headaches, hunger pains, weakness or irritability and lost on average a pound a day.

By the 1970s, hCG was the most widely administered obesity medication in the United States, but it was only approved by the FDA as a fertility drug. So in 1976, the Federal Trade Commission ordered Dr. Simeons to stop claiming his hCG program was safe or approved by the FDA for weight control. The order did not stop the clinics from using hCG. It just required that patients be informed in writing the following:

"HCG has not been demonstrated to be an effective adjunctive therapy in the treatment of obesity. There is no substantial evidence that it increases weight loss beyond that resulting from caloric restriction, that it causes a more attractive or "normal" distribution of fat or that it decreases the hunger and discomfort associated with calorie-restricted diets."

Dr. Simeons originally put his patients on a strict 500 calorie diet with very tight controls on exactly which foods could be used. Dr. Simeons prohibited his patients from use of regular medications prescribed by their physician, however, because he required his patients to see him every day, he could resume a specific medication if needed. His patients were not allowed to eat breakfast or take any vitamins except for coral calcium. They could only take hCG by intramuscular injection.

The new 800 calorie hCG diet protocol suggests a daily calorie intake between 550-800 which has been found to be more tolerable, much safer, and has produced similar weight loss results. The body is technically "starving" if a less than 800 calorie diet has been consumed for the day. It is suggested to stay between 725-750 calories daily to prevent going above the 800 daily limit. This increase in calories has enabled my patients to complete the entire 6 weeks with reduced complaints of hunger, weakness, and headaches. The additional calories added to the protocol were mostly obtained from adding more protein sources providing 3 major benefits. Protein:

1. Assists in preserving lean muscle mass
2. Increases fat burning
3. Helps curb appetite by up to 40 % throughout the day

I have found that combining the following guidelines will result in maximizing your success:

1. Stay-below 800 calories
2. Higher protein intake compared to the original (increase your intake of protein)
3. Follow the food guide provided

4. Take a daily whole-food multi-vitamin/mineral and suggested supplements

5. Eat breakfast and snacks

6. Continuing all prescription medications

7. Participate in light cardio aerobic exercise or physical activity for 30 minutes daily

8. Drink half your body weight in ounces daily

9. Have good coaching support

10. Maintain an accurate daily food journal

11. Stay POP and you will DROP. (POP-Perfect on Protocol)

The thousands of patients I have coached have successfully lost weight while taking hCG without the effects of feeling tired and hungry. In addition, many have reported an increase in energy and motivation. Most women who carefully follow the new hCG Diet Protocol have lost, on average, a half a pound per day or 20 to 35 pounds in 40 days. Men who carefully follow the new 800 hCG Diet Protocol tend to lose more, about a pound per day or 35 to 45 pounds.

As a licensed health care professional, I feel it is imperative to educate the hCG dieter on how to lose weight safely while on the hCG diet or any restricted-calorie weight loss plan. Modern medicine and nutritional information has vastly improved since the 1950's when the original protocol was first discovered. My goal is for you to learn why a healthier approach to the original protocol will have a positive effect on your body's response to weight loss and assist in the prevention of weight-related diseases.

Please make sure you have approval from your physician before beginning any restricted-calorie diet.

hCG Weight Loss Clinical Studies

Successful Weight Loss Intervention Using a Modified hCG Diet

In 2010, the President of the ASBP performed a 6-week successful clinical study on a modified 800 calorie hCG diet with the use of sublingual Rx hCG hormone. 19 hCG patients were compared with 19 patients using an 800 calorie daily meal replacement diet without hCG. "**Results**: The modified hCG diet patients lost an average of 19.84 lbs in 6 weeks, whereas the meal replacement patients lost 14.75 lbs. The average decrease in BMI in the hCG group was 3.18 and 2.48 in the meal replacement group." **Conclusion**: "Sublingual hCG appeared to be significantly better in weight loss than a similar meal replacement diet of comparable protein and calorie composition. The results revealed a relatively rapid weight loss in 6 weeks with preservation of lean body mass. Furthermore, it appears that this approach could have a benefit to the patients in that they demonstrated reduced usage of controlled substances for appetite. As this study revealed that sublingual hCG with a modified diet was beneficial to patients in assisting them with weight loss..."

To view the full clinical trial, please visit **http://www.weightshop.net/documents/Bryman%20HCG%20Article.pdf**

American Journal of Clinical Nutrition

www.ajcn.org and the American Society of Bariatric Physicians Research Council, 333 West Hampden Avenue, Englewood, Colorado 80110

Effect of human chorionic gonadotrophin on weight loss, hunger, and feeling of well-being

Authored by:

W. L. Asher, MD and Harold W. Harper, MD

Twenty female patients on 500- to 550- kcal diets receiving daily injections of 125 IU of human chorionic gonadotrophin (hCG) were compared with 20 female patients on 500- to 550-kcal diets receiving placebo injections. Patients in both groups were instructed to return for daily injections 6 days each week for a total of 36 injections (unless desired weight was achieved prior to this). The hCG group lost significantly more mean weight, had a significantly greater mean weight loss per injection, and lost a significantly greater mean percentage of their starting weight. The percentage of affirmative daily patient responses indicating "little or no hunger" and "feeling good to excellent" was significantly greater in the HCG group than in the placebo group. Additional investigation of the influence of hCG on weight loss, hunger, and well-being seems indicated.

American Journal of Clinical Nutrition, Vol. 26, 211-218, Copyright © 1973 by the American Society for Clinical Nutrition, Inc.

REVISED 800 CALORIE PROTOCOL LCD	"Original" Dr. Simeons PROTOCOL VLCD
550-800 calories daily – LCD - Low Calorie Diet	500 calories daily – VLCD - Very Low Calorie Diet
Eat breakfast to include 1 protein and fruit serving	No breakfast (optional fruit serving only)
Effectively an LCD; is safer than the original	Effectively a VLCD mandating closer supervision
More selection of green vegetables, higher protein content and additional fruit serving	Limited food choices
Multi-vitamin/minerals highly suggested	No vitamins except calcium
Take all medications prescribed by your MD	Suggested to stop all medications
hCG available in sublingual form and sub-Q injectable	Dr. Simeons gave his patients only intramuscular injections

Detailed hCG Diet Book that is an exceptional educational tool	Hard to understand pamphlet "Pounds and Inches" written 50 years ago, very confusing to most
Updated Phase 3 that ensures a successful stabilization	Phase 3 is vague and confusing to most
Recipes for Phases 2-3 meals	Limited list of food to prepare
Products in protocol are easy to find at stores	Some products are difficult to find at stores.

Chapter 1

hCG Controversy: 500 VS 800

Everyone knows that the biggest scrutiny with the Dr. Simeon's original is the 500 calories. Anyone can lose weight eating just 500 calories, right? The hCG diet has been very controversial over the last 50+ years, yet it keeps coming back, and it keeps providing results *when done correctly*. This is something that can't be ignored, yet the medical community will not consider a 500 calorie diet, but 800 calories... this is where the controversy within controversy comes in.

A lot of dieters have the mentality, "if it ain't broke, don't fix it," but what if something isn't broken, but there is a way to make it better? Times have changed! Look at all of our advancements in medicine, technology, and research abilities. It is changing exponentially.

I had the good fortune of meeting Candice Ekberg, B.S. ESS, AEMT and personal fitness trainer, who was featured on a popular television talk show last year touting her weight loss on the hCG diet. I challenged Candice to try the 800 Calorie Protocol to see for herself that the updated version delivers the same level of success as the original but is now more comfortable and most of all, safer than ever. Candice intentionally gained weight so she would be able to compare the 500 VS 800, pound for pound and inch by inch. The results are most impressive.

Before and after results of hCG Diet 800 Calorie Diet in July 2011:

6/27/11 – Before	Sonia E Russell LPN 800 Calorie	7/19/11 – After
43"	Shoulders	42.5" = -0.5
36.5"	Chest	36" = -0.5
31"	Waist(narrowest)	28.5" = -2.5
36.75"	Abdomen(at BB)	33.5" = -3.25
39.5"	Hip(widest)	37.5" = -2.0
23.75"	Thigh(thickest)	22.5" = -1.25
14.75"	Calve	14.25" = -0.5
12.5"	Bicep	11.75" = -0.75
23.1%	Hand held BIA	**18.8% = -4.3%**
19.05%	4 site Lange Caliper	14.23% = -4.82%
BL 160.5	Weight – **Final 150.1**	BL = – 10.4
AL 165.5		AL = – 15.4
	Inches Lost	**11.25" total, -9" off W, H, A, T**

*Before Load/After Load

Candice kept all of her data from previous rounds.

Before and after Dr. Simeon's 500 calorie in January 2011

1/4/11 – Before	Dr. Simeon's 500 calorie	1/28/11 – After
43.5″	Shoulders	42.25″ = .75″
37″	Chest	36″ = -1.0″
30.75″	Waist(narrowest)	29.5″ = -1.25″
35.5″	Abdomen(at BB)	34.5″ = -1.0″
39.5″	Hip(widest)	38.25″ = -.75″
23.25″	Thigh(thickest)	23″ = -0.25″
14.75″	Calve	14.25″ = -0.5
12.25″	Bicep	12″ = -0.25
22.1%	Hand BIA	**19.8% = -2.2%**
BL 160.3	Weight – **152.5**	
AL 166.6		
	Inches Lost	-5.5" total, -3.25" off *W, H, A, T

*Before Load/After Load *Waist, Hip, Ab, Thigh

Side by Side comparison of Candice's results with Sonia E Russell's 800 Calorie Protocol VS. Dr. Simeon's 500 Calorie Protocol

	Russell's 800 – 23 days	Simeon's 500 – 23 days
Shoulders	42.5″ -0.5	42.25″ -.75
Chest	36″ -0.5	36″ -1.0
Waist	28.5″ -2.5	29.5″ -1.25
Abdomen	33.5″ -3.25	34.5″ - 1.0
Hips	37.5″ -2.0	38.25″ - .75
Thigh	22.5″ -1.25	23″ - .25
Calve	14.5″ -.5	14.25″ -.25
Bicep	11.75″ -.75	12″ -.25
Total Inches Lost	-11.25″ – 9″ off W, H, A, T	- 5.5″ – 3.25″ off W, H, A, T
BIA	23.1->18.8% – 4.3%	22.1% -> 19.8% -2.2%
4 site caliper	19.05% -> 14.23% -4.82%	didn't use calipers
Weight	BL 160.5/AL 165.5	BL 160.3/AL 166.6
	Final – 150.1 = -10.4BL, – 15.4AL	Final – 152.5 = -7.8BL, -13.8AL

By eating 800 calories instead of 500, including breakfast, more protein, adding an extra fruit, and supplementing, she was able to lose 5.75″ more inches and 2.6 more pounds (pre-load), 1.6 more than after loading. But what is more important than the scale itself is the QUALITY of those pounds. She was able to lose **2.1% MORE BODY FAT** than she did with the 500. The best part about this all is that she felt great. Candice explained that she only experienced one day of hunger while on the 800 VLCD, whereas on the 500 she felt as if she was starving for 2 full weeks. She also experienced intermittent headaches and fatigue on the 500, which she did not experience on the 800.

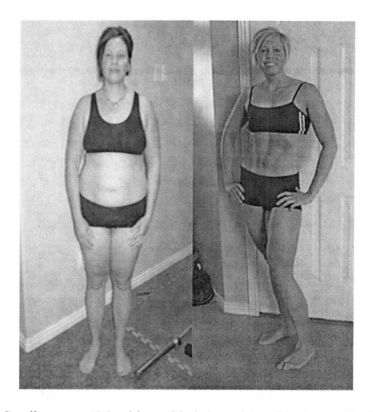

Candice says, "My skin and hair have been fabulous! All of my previous rounds, my hands and knuckles would get so dry due to not being able to use lotion. I would also get ashy on my legs. I've gone through a whole bottle of Aveeno lotion in a round before. This round, the only time I put it on was after I showered or washed my hands. Even my heels are great! They have always been prone to cracking and peeling during the summer when I wear sandals all the time. My hair normally grows super slow and I can go 6-8 weeks without a cut or color, but I already have bad root growth after 5 weeks... this is actually kind of a pain! I attribute these differences to supplements. Energy wise, I feel great! I was even able to workout at a light to moderate rate. I really lagged on the 500, and would have days where I didn't want to do anything but sit... not this time."

Candice Ekberg

Testimonials

"The HCG Diet 800 Calorie Protocol is amazing. I've dropped 70 pounds so far. I've never been able to lose more than 25 pounds on any other diet program I've tried (and I've tried A LOT of them over the last 25 years!) Eventually, I lost all hope of successful weight loss. Then I discovered hCG. For the first time ever, I believe I not only have a real shot at taking off my excess weight but also keeping it off.

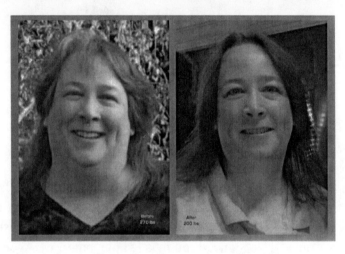

Blood tests confirm major internal improvements:

A1c is down from 5.9 to 5.4
Fasting glucose down from 117 to 87
Fasting insulin down from 9.9 to 3.4 (wow!!)

That means no more pre-diabetes, no more impaired fasting glucose, and no more insulin resistance. Not only that, my coronary panel has shown improvements as well,,,

Cholesterol total down from 194 to 176
Triglycerides down from 153 to 114
CRP/Cardio down from 1.6 to 0.6

This officially moves me from the 'moderate' risk of heart disease category to the 'low' risk category.

The HCG Diet 800 Calorie Protocol has worked miracles for me!"

Margaret Downey

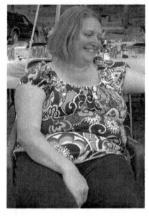

"Growing up, I had always been very active and never overweight. I kept active in soccer & track and in college I started distance running. I had the typical "Freshman 15" creep on but still managed to be active enough to be considered "normal." Slowly the 15 extra pounds turned into 25. After 3 pregnancies, 2 moves and about 500 Big Macs, I found that I had ballooned up over 100 lbs. At 5'7", 265 lbs. was not what I wanted to be carrying around. I set out determined to find a way to take the weight off. I tried everything … name brand diets, pills, exercise, ads from infomercials that promised if you sprinkled this on your food you would lose weight, limiting carbs, limiting fat, eating only protein … you name it, I tried it! I would lose on some but usually regained what I had lost.

It was just after my youngest child turned 1 year old that I got my wake-up call. My husband found out that he would be working out of town in Hawaii (of all places.) Even just the thought of putting on a swim suit and taking my boys to the beach repulsed me. Of course that is when I ran across my "before" picture. (One of the few that I had allowed to be taken of me because I often hid from cameras as I never liked what I saw.) Sitting on the floor with that picture, I cried. I saw my father in that picture. He was the rock and stability in my life and passed away at the age of 52. He was diagnosed with diabetes in his 30s and by the time he was 51 had his leg amputated because of the lack of care of his diabetes. Three months after his amputation, a blood clot broke free and took my father. I cried because I KNEW that my road was starting to merge with his. Knowing that I would be turning 40 in the next couple years (I was 38 at the time) I HAD to do something to change the course my life was headed on. I did NOT want to leave my kids early as my father had.

After a month of researching online, I downloaded a copy of "Pounds & Inches" by Dr. Simeons to start my journey. I weighed 224 when I began in December of 2010. It truly was a struggle as I really didn't know what I was doing and had to learn a lot of things the hard way. (Like you can't take the easy way and just eat chicken luncheon meat.) I found several groups online that had support, but mostly just fellow dieters like myself that really didn't know what they were doing either.

One day in March 2011, I noted a post from someone I had friended along the way. A nurse from Florida, named Sonia, had posted a challenge on her page asking questions about the hCG diet that I actually knew the answer too. This was the start of a friendship that was to change my life forever. On the 500 calorie diet, I experienced a lot of hair loss. I had lost about 40 lbs. by then and knew I didn't want to quit, but I also didn't want to be bald. I sent a message to this nurse and this began our conversations about nutrition, vitamins and the 800 caloric protocol.

I am pretty set in my ways and when something works, I don't really want to mess with it. It wasn't until my 4th round that I decided to give the 800 calorie protocol a try.

I knew I was getting close to goal and was worried that it would be more difficult to lose as I got closer. I also was still concerned about hair loss. This was the best decision I made on the diet. Not only did I no longer have issues with hair loss, but I wasn't hungry like before and found that I had way more energy. (Which is a good thing when you are chasing 3 boys under the age of 5 years old around.) It was also during this round that we ended up moving half way across the country for a new job. Yes, I MOVED in P2. So the amazing thing about all 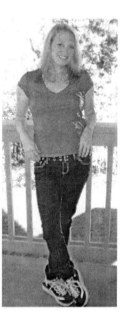 this was that I lost more weight than any of my other 500 rounds.

> R1= -16.6 lbs. in 40 days (8% of my body weight)
> R2= -19.4 lbs. in 35 days (10% of my body weight)
> R3= -21.8 lbs. in 35 days (12% of my body weight)
> R4= -25.6 lbs. in 40 days (16% of my body weight)
> **– this was my 800 Calorie Protocol round**

Now sitting 125 lbs. down from my heaviest weight, I'm thankful for all the changes that hCG and Sonia's protocol have brought to my life. I can race my boy's home from school and not feel like I'm dying. I can sit in a chair with all three boys and not worry that the chair will break. My family is learning to eat vegetables and understand the importance of healthy food. Most important, I know I have gained back years to watch my children grow and hopefully grandchildren and great-grandchildren."

Melissa

"My Journey to Health"

"In the 32 years since I graduated from college I have gained (and occasionally lost) about 110 pounds. I was 150 in college at 5'9" and that was great. But ever since I had struggled to keep there and battled an insatiable appetite and I was never "full" even when my stomach was stuffed. I found myself at 267 pounds in the summer of 2010. Eating from stress and boredom had landed me in pre-diabetes with danger-zone numbers for heart disease and herniated disks resulting in nerve damage. I stumbled across hCG in the summer of 2010. I had just spent a week mourning the loss of my older brother to heart disease, and his doctor suggested I try to regain my health through hCG.

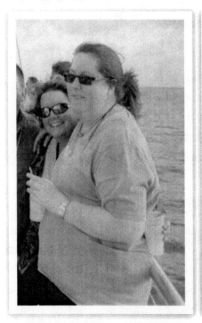 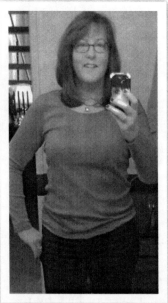

Before: 267 pounds
After: 184 pounds (4 rounds)

I started my first round on September 1, 2010 following the protocol of Dr. A.T.W. Simeons. In 30 days I shed 30 pounds. A miracle! I stabilized well and stayed even through the holiday parties and travel. I did round 2 in January 2011 and lost 20 pounds in 25 days. Round 3 in March was 18 pounds in 30 days. In this round I began to have considerable hair loss. I have really thick hair, but it was still worrisome. I wondered what else could be resulting from the hCG and the 500 calorie protocol. I took a long break and went on 4 vacations over 4 months. I gained back the 18 pounds lost in Round 3.

When I was ready to do my 4th round, I read about the 800 calorie protocol on Candice Ekberg's blog comparing her results in the two protocols. She convinced me that the 800 calorie approach was healthier AND just as rapid in the weight loss. So I gave it a try. My 4th round was 45 days and I dropped 33 pounds! I had no hair loss, no hunger and it was so very easy to stick to the protocol. I averaged 650 calories a day. This round brought my weight to 183 pounds as of Sept 15, 2011. The stabilization of that weight in P3 has been truly amazing. By following the strict P3 guidelines, I stayed 2 pounds under my Last Dose Weight for 4 weeks. And then slowly added in regular foods – sprouted grain breads, nuts, cheeses and have maintained that weight for 8 weeks. I can hardly wait to do my final round in January 2012 to get to my goal weight of 165 pounds. A normal BMI will be a welcome state for my 54th year!"

As of June 2012, Anne has maintained her weight at 130 pounds.

Anne

"I was heavy most of my life and always the overweight girl. My Mom and Dad would say, "oh you are just stocky but you are healthy". I have struggled with my weight from the moment I was born. I weighed 11 pounds and 8 ½ ounces and 22 ¾ inch long. So I have literally had to struggle with weight issues from the moment I was born and I am 48 years old now. I have been on all kinds of diets all my life. I would lose the same 25 pounds about twenty different times in my life.

My life as a whole is great; I have a loving husband of 25 years, two great kids and 3 grandkids. They have always been my life. I have always done for everyone else. If anyone needed me I was there. Over the course of the last 14 years now I steadily put on weight. I got to a point in my life and I remember it very clearly, my husband and I talked about it even. We talked about how much weight we both have gained. And we both said," well I guess that is life, this is what happens when you get older". We both fell into the pattern of as long as we are this way and we don't gain anymore we will be ok. We actually had this conversation and convinced ourselves it was ok to be overweight. Until Last year it wasn't ok anymore.

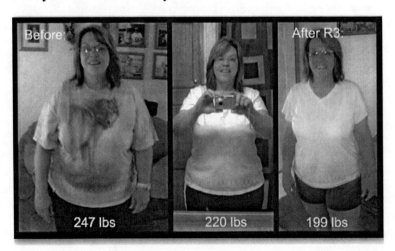

I was getting really sick all the time, I noticed I started gaining weight and was short of breath. I could hardly walk without hurting. I noticed people were starting to stare at me when I ate or when I went to a restaurant ordering food or buying clothes. I would hear comments from people that were not so nice. But I tried to ignore them and pretend they weren't talking about me.

I decided one day I would stop smoking and then my next goal was going to lose weight. Well I accomplished the stop smoking, I smoked for 25 years. That was difficult in itself, but I did it. And wouldn't you know it there was more weight coming on. Twenty-five more pounds. I thought wow; my husband is going to leave me if I keep this up. Then about 4 months later I got really sick and was rushed to the Emergency room. They did all kinds of test, ultra sounds, blood work, x-rays. Come to find out that the awful pain that I was having would result in needing a complete hysterectomy. My doctor also diagnosed me with Hypothyroidism which explains some of the weight gain. I had the surgery, went through recovery and my medication was monitored for my thyroid. A couple months went by and it is Christmas. I had gained some more weight. Now I am seeing pictures of myself, crying my eyes out. I couldn't lose the weight no matter what I did. The sarcasm and comments from strangers increased the more my weight increased. I went home most nights and cried. You see I am an EMT and I help people like myself every day. I couldn't seem to help myself though. Until one day in March, I did some research on the Internet. There was a diet that I had never heard of. Believe me when I say I have tried them all and none had worked. I found hCG and I asked my friends if they had heard about this diet. Some had, but didn't know too much about it. Well I found a group on Facebook that did. By the end of April I ordered my first hCG pellets. Started my very first round on May 1st

I never weighed myself at home in about 5 months. I always depended on the doctor's office to weigh me, and my last visit was before Christmas. My beginning weight on May 1st was 247.4. I know at one time I was heavier than that. You see I started going to the gym in January and lost some weight before I started hCG but I don't know how much it was. At this time I had lost 62 pounds. I had 25-35 more pounds to lose. I can say with certainty that if I wouldn't have found hCG I would be a lot heavier then I was. I was also borderline Diabetic and developing heart and lung problems. HCG has saved my life. I know longer pre-diabetic or have heart problems. I haven't had any lung problems in 7 months and no more episodes of shortness of breath. Finally now I can be a role model for my patients. And most of all I can be there for my family and my grandkids. I will be able to live long enough to watch them grow up. They can see that they have a grandmother that is healthy and able to run and play. I can say I am healthier now than I have been in the last 10 years. I am so thankful for hCG and Sonia's Protocol. It works! I am looking so forward to reaching my goal and having a life time of health by maintaining my goal weight."

Colleen

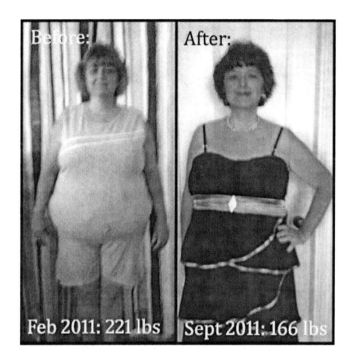

Before: After:

Feb 2011: 221 lbs Sept 2011: 166 lbs

"I found a group online who supported the 500 calorie protocol and did 2 rounds on it. The thing was I was losing weight but I was also suffering. I am a school bus driver and I was always tired, sometimes weak and would have to go to bed in between my school runs. At the end of the second round my hair was falling out. I came across Sonia Russell's site on the 800 calorie protocol and read the posts daily. I joined in with my limited knowledge and then made a decision to do my 3rd round with the 800. I was nervous because I lost a good amount of weight with the 500 and was not convinced I could with 800. Sonia offered to guide me through so I began. I noticed immediately a difference. Because she recommends supplements, my energy levels stayed up....plus we ate breakfast daily...no weakness. I wasn't hungry and it was easier to stay focused. I enjoyed the entire 40 days and lost 19 lbs. I would have lost more but I stalled at first trying to figure things out. It convinced me that doing this protocol was a healthier way to lose weight and I am currently on my 4th round doing 800. I would not do 500 again. Thanks to Sonia and the doctors who researched this. Everyone looks at me amazed because I have lost all together 59 lbs. and I am 53 years old and Hypothyroid. My doctor said I was heading toward fatty liver disease and my latest liver test came back normal. Also my cholesterol went from 256 to 160.I would encourage anyone who wants to lose weight to get their blood work done before they start and work along with your doctor. My doctor loves the fact the weight is coming off and it is the obesity today that is killing people. Finally, there is a safe way to lose weight and maintain it."

Betty

"I grew up with a very addictive personality. I am a recovered alcoholic of 13 years and ended up with alcohol induced liver cirrhosis at age 25. I quit smoking a year ago due to chronic lung infections and asthma caused by smoking. All my life I turned to food. It became my worst addiction to date. It caused me to spiral out of control many times in my life during times of stress and just making poor choices. I am an emotional eater. I ended up at 205lbs, and at 5 foot 2, that extra weight was killing me. I had to quit the job that I love as store manager for a pet store chain, and take stress leave. I had such a hard time even putting on socks and shoes. I could barely brace myself to get up off the floor and climbing up stairs was almost impossible. At age 38, I was so embarrassed and humiliated with myself that I ended up this way by my own doing. I had so much abnormal fat around my mid-section and my joints ached. I knew I was killing myself slowly but surely. I was in a lot of pain due to being obese. I became isolated and bed ridden.

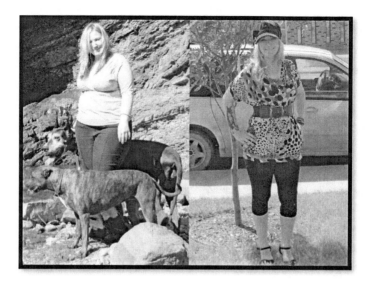

My Great Dane, Justice, who was a senior and at the end of her life, was severely obese herself. She ended up with osteoarthritis in her back hip due to her weight. She fell daily, and at 165lbs herself, I could literally not help her up off the floor. I was too fat. I blamed myself for her ailment, went into a depression and saw no way out. I was suicidal for letting myself get so out of control. I felt like I failed my big girl and failed myself. One day I was on the computer and came across hCG through a friend that also had Great Danes. I read the protocol and got a glimmer of hope! I promised Justice, that I would get help for myself so I could help her. HCG came into my life in September of 2011 and I started my journey. I managed to lose 40lbs through hCG by the time Justice died. It took me 2 rounds of 40 days on the protocol! I was able to get her up off the floor with ease. Even after that first 10 lbs. I lost, everything seemed so much easier! I couldn't believe how fast it came off, how easy it was to stick to the protocol and eat clean, wholesome foods. The best part, I had no hunger and so much more energy! I even noticed my moods were getting better and I was sleeping soundly at night for the first time in months. Justice`s last months on earth with me

were her best, as I was able to do so many more things for
her due to my rapid weight loss. She was happy and so was
I for the first time in years! I did not fail her after all. After
she died, I decided to continue on with hCG and help as
many people as I could by sharing my story and knowledge
on the protocol. Justice was my inspiration, as without her
being so sick, I don't believe I would have done anything
about my weight. I was desperate back then, and in my
desperation, I did what seemed to be impossible at the time,
possible!

I have now completed 4 rounds. I have lost 65lbs through
Sonia's hCG protocol! These books have been a true
godsend for me and I will continue to my goal weight
following these books. I am just a few lbs. away from my
healthy BMI of 136lbs. I can't believe just a short time ago
I was topping the scales at 205lbs! I have yo yo'd my whole
life, going as high as 247lbs with my lowest weight of
115lbs and everything in between. I have tried several
popular diets with no success at all. I also spent thousands
of dollars on these diets. I realize now, since following the
hCG protocol, it's the sugar and starch that is allowed in
other diets that have always caused a problem for me. Any
bit of starch at all, spirals me out of control. Portion control
on any diet that allowed starch was my biggest failure.

I saved a lot of money following the hCG protocol because
I was able to buy my own food and spend a fraction on
drops, than what I would have spent going to other diet
centers. The support by others doing this protocol has been
phenomenal! I have never felt so motivated and inspired
before, like I have in this community.

The hCG protocol taught me how to grocery shop for
wholesome foods, and how to cook healthy for myself. I no
longer worry about yo-yo dieting. I have been able to

master portion control for the first time in my life! I even addressed my emotional eating while on hCG, and find solace in wholesome foods for comfort. I am completely off sugar now and diet soda thanks to this protocol. I will never have to go up and down in my weight again. I have no more excuses! I know how to keep myself stabilized because of this protocol. I truly believe that my life has been saved because of hCG and these guides. My doctor ran blood work on me since my huge loss in weight, and I am so healthy! I am in the best shape I have been in years! Just a short time ago, I could barely walk up stairs, now I can walk and run in intervals, 10km's! I feel amazing! My next goal is to get back on skis! I will get there, thanks to hCG!"

Krista

"The 800 Calorie Protocol and hCG have given me back my life!"

"Let me start by saying in 2006 I married the man of my dreams. I wore a size 7 wedding dress, weighing in at 135 pounds (I'm 5 ft. 2 in). We were very active. We mountain-biked, we roller-bladed, we loved camping and any type of active outdoor activity.

After 2 years, I became very ill. We went from doctor to doctor with no answer, though we did have one tell me I was allergic to sodium and to get off every form of salt. Soon after that I starting to forget things like my children's birthdays, my address, and my phone number. I could no longer work or go anywhere by myself because I wouldn't be able to find my way home. I started sleeping 14 hours a day. I also began to put on weight at a very alarming rate. I gained 60 pounds the first year, then 20 to 30 pounds every year after that. I remember feeling my flesh ripping that last year. It was such a horrible and hopeless feeling. I was eventually told I had the worst case of fibromyalgia this one doctor had ever seen and was put on a lot of medications.

In the spring of 2009, I found an excellent doctor who diagnosed me with a severe hypothyroid issue. He informed my husband and I that the lack of sodium and all the medication from the misdiagnosis of fibromyalgia had shut down my thyroid and I was going into a Myxedema coma, that one day soon he would have come home and found me dead in the bed had this not been discovered when it was. The doctor assured me that the weight gain was from the non-functioning thyroid and put me on a serious high dose of thyroid medication and told me the weight would melt off as I began to feel better. I did begin to feel better fast and I began to get up and move. I started walking 2 miles a day, three days a week, with no weight loss results. I changed my diet and still nothing. I had 2 jawbone surgeries in the summer of 2009 and could not eat anything but somehow managed to gain 3 pounds. I knew then that my metabolism had shut down. I kept trying everything to lose with no results.

In the summer of 2010, I ruptured the discs in my lower back and the doctor told me to get the weight off or I would be looking at steel rods. I did some brief research on hCG and ordered it from India. I didn't even know what I was getting. I did the injections and lost 21 pounds in 21 days. Eureka! I found gold. The owners of the company that I work for did more research and discovered hCG drops. Since I do not like needles, I decided to try it. That round I lost 23 pounds in 21 days. That was it. I was hooked. After a few rounds … some good, some bad … I met an awesome lady on a sweet support group who began to talk to me about the 800 protocol. I was on my fifth round by then (I was doing short 21 day rounds). She asked me if I would like to try the 800 Calorie hCG Protocol and I thought, "Why not? I will try anything once." So, I did, and lost 26 pounds in 21 days. The whole time I felt amazing, had great energy and mental clarity, and from that moment on I knew I found the right combination for me. I have done 5 rounds on the 500 and 4 rounds on the 800. I will not ever do another 500 again."

Bj Brooks

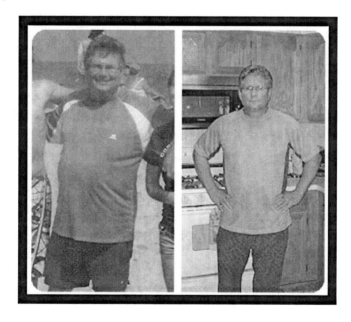

"I thought you would like to know about my results from following the protocol.

BEFORE | AFTER

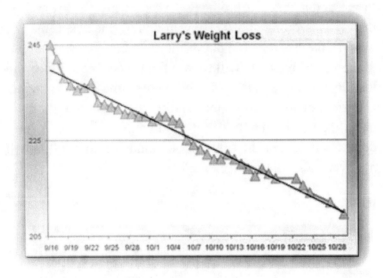

"I used an electronic scale which is capable of measuring each. As you can see, I lost almost 36 pounds, the bulk of which was fat! I had no loss of muscle by percent of body weight, and actually increased my hydration significantly. Amazing! Also, my energy levels are through the roof. I'm back to playing competitive tennis, I've been off of all medications for over three months - I no longer suffer from acid reflux/chronic heartburn, depression, high blood pressure."

Larry

"I started on July 12, 2007 weighing at 241 pounds now today I weigh 159 pounds. That is 82 pounds! I'm 38 and have not weighed 159 since I was a sophomore in high school. I did 3 rounds of HCG and finished in April 2008. To date I fluctuate between 158 and 162 pounds. I have tried most of the weight loss programs out there and none compares to this. I tell everybody about it and 3 of my friends have started it now. My life has never been so great!"

Brian

"I made it all the way through Phase II including the 3-day weaning period of coming off the injections. I'm proud to say I did not cheat even a teeny bit the entire time, (and I have tried many diets, believe me). My scale consistently showed an average loss of one-half pound per day all the way to the last day of injections. On the last day of my injections, I weighed 139.8 pounds. Before the first injection I weighed 166.8. So my total Phase II weight loss was 27 pounds!!!! I can't thank you enough for everything. My weight has stabilized at 138 and I'm a happy girl! Not bad for a 51 year old."

Anita

"I completed my six weeks round of hCG and completed the three week maintenance with tremendous results. I am now in Phase 4 which is maintaining your weight for the rest of your life. I was on a 7 day cruise last week and am probably the only person that came back having LOST a pound vs. gaining any weight. This program really does work."

Dru

"How I Kept the Weight Off for 2 Years"

"It has been two years since I took hCG and happy to say I have managed to keep off the weight.

I was a tiny little thing in high school, a size 2. But I had three kids and I went up to a size 10, 155 pounds. I know that doesn't sound awful, but I felt uncomfortable. My body wasn't made to be that size.

I tried exercising and watching what I ate but I didn't lose much weight. I read about hCG in a book and decided to try it.

The first four days were the roughest. But once I started to lose the weight, it kept me going. By the time I finished phase 1, I was down 25 pounds.

But then in phase 3, I neglected to follow the diet instructions. You're supposed to follow a strict diet at this point so you can reset your metabolism and lock in your weight. No sugars. No carbs. Only certain fruits, vegetables and proteins.

I screwed up. I ate sauces and nuts with salt. I put 10 pounds back on.

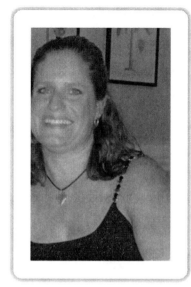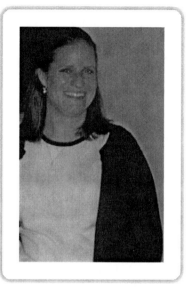

So I did a second round of hCG and this time, I lost 25 pounds and I was careful to follow the diet in its entirety.

I can't tell you how happy it made me feel to lose this weight. I put a size 2 on and I wanted to scream. I was so excited and I felt better.

It has been two years since I lost the weight and it hasn't been that hard to keep it off. This diet changed the way I view food. For 60 days, I had no sugars or carbs. When I stopped the diet, I wasn't craving those types of foods as much.

I do eat carbs and desserts now. In fact, I eat dessert maybe once a week.

But I pay attention to what I eat the rest of the week. If I know I'm going to go out and have Margaritas on a Friday night, I'm going to work for it during the week. Basically I pay the piper.

And when I eat carbs, I watch which ones I eat. I'll eat brown rice and multi-grain bread and wheat pasta. And I'll only have them like once a day. I avoid hydrogenated oils and items that have high fructose corn syrup and white flour. I no longer drink Diet Coke.

And I'm not a couch potato. I do two spin classes a week. I walk a lot and run once a week.

Lots of people ask me my secret and I when I tell them about hCG, they are surprised. But now some of my friends are trying it and having success also.

Now that I'm slimmer, I feel really good about myself. I'm 41 years old but I feel much younger. It's so nice to have your husband say, "oh my gosh, you look like you did when I first met you!

I avoided keeping photos of myself before I lost the weight so these were the only ones that I could find. Now, I enjoy having my picture taken!"

Gigi English

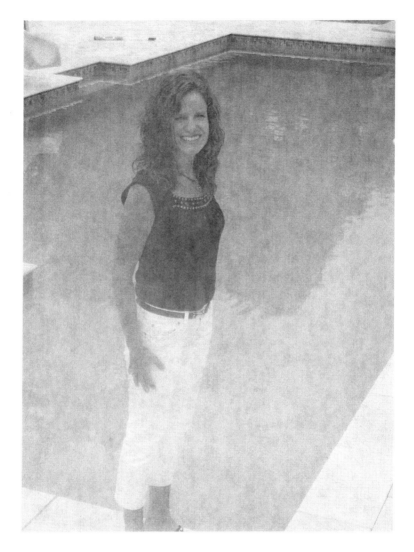

Gigi 2 years later!

Chapter 2

The Obesity Epidemic

The United States is currently the heaviest nation in the world. The health consequences of this are enormous. The diseases associated with weight gain and obesity are well known and include the following:

- Heart disease
- Diabetes type 2
- Osteoarthritis
- High blood pressure
- Gallbladder disease
- Breast cancer
- Endometrial cancer
- Colon cancer

The risk of worsening illness (morbidity) increases as weight increases for the following conditions:

- Respiratory problems
- Cancers of the uterus, breast, prostate, and colon
- Sleep apnea
- Infertility
- Stress incontinence
- Psychological problems including depression

The good news is that by decreasing your weight by just by 10% you will enjoy a significant improvement in your health. The hCG Diet will help you attain the goal of lowering your weight and reducing your risk of disease or death due to obesity–related illness. You will not only look better but feel better, and you can't beat that.

Obesity

- 68% of Americans (over 160 million people) are overweight or obese, and the numbers continue to increase

- The current economic situation results in less expensive and more fattening foods consumed for example; fast-foods, processed foods, canned foods, and high fructose corn syrup.

- Most diets fail in the long run

- Most people do not maintain their weight loss

Why Most Diets May Fail?

- Most diets may result in a loss of lean muscle which can slow down metabolism resulting in excessive weight gain. Most of the time the patient will gain their weight back and often much more!

- Emotional / behavioral eating caused by stress.

- Medical science has proven that those who are overweight/obese, diabetics, and those with thyroid disease are Leptin resistant.

What is Leptin Resistance?

Leptin is a hormone made in your fat cells and is needed to control metabolism and hunger. Leptin resistance occurs when the hypothalamus gland in the brain is unable to receive a signal that you are full, thus chronic weight gain occurs. Highly processed sugary foods such as High Fructose Corn

Syrup cause the pancreas to produce large levels of Insulin. Elevated Insulin levels cause fat storage which leads to Leptin resistance and facilitates chronic weight gain.

Long Term Factors in Weight Loss/Gain

1) Slower Metabolism

The more you diet, the harder it is to lose weight. Most weight loss programs result in a loss of lean muscle which may slow metabolism. Most of the time the patient will gain their weight back and more!

2) Aging –Declining Hormones

As we age, our hormone levels naturally decline as well as our metabolism. This is significant with menopausal women that most often complain of the "menopausal extra 30 pounds". The hormones of youth (ex. Testosterone, Estrogen, Progesterone, Growth Hormone, DHEA) also decrease and/or become imbalanced, thus weight gain ensues.

3) Prolonged Stress

The hormone Cortisol increases with stress and may cause the body to store fat. High levels of Cortisol may cause insulin levels to rise, predisposing the patient to Diabetes. Stress may also drive down DHEA, a hormone produced by the Adrenal Glands that assists in endocrine function.

4) Life style

Poor eating habits and lack of exercise

5) Health Status

Disease and medications

6) Genetics

Thyroid disease and many other metabolic conditions

7) Emotional/Behavioral issues (stress, depression, and anxiety)

Stress elevates Cortisol levels and depression may lead to overeating

8) Skipping Breakfast

People that skip breakfast are **450%** more likely to become overweight and obese

9) Hunger

The body will store fat if it is not properly nourished. The hormone Ghrelin, produced in the gastro-intestinal tract rises when you are hungry for prolonged periods, which facilitates the storage of fat.

Rollercoaster Dieting/Yo-Yo Dieting

Starvation diets - VLCD (very low calorie diets) and LCD (low calorie diets) without hCG may cause a loss of lean muscle that may result in a slower metabolism.

■ These diets typically fail and all the weight lost is gained back plus more!

- A slower metabolism may make it harder and harder to lose weight.

- Fat cell size and number increase with weight gain. Fat cell size will only decrease when you lose weight. The more you Yo-Yo diet, the more fat cells will multiply so this is why it gets tougher and tougher to lose weight the more a person diets.

Diets that May Cause Loss of Muscle

- Starvation and Ketosis Dieting

- VLCD's & LCD's - Diets less than 800 calories daily

- Eating less than 3 meals per day

What is HCG?

- Human Chorionic Gonadotropin is a glycoprotein hormone produced by the placenta in pregnancy that stimulates production of progesterone, allowing the uterus to sustain a growing fetus.

- Hormone that indicates pregnancy (positive when pregnant).

- The hCG hormone protects and nourishes the fetus by delivering caloric nutrition to the placenta by obtaining nutrition from the mother.

- For weight loss, prescribed off label, hCG is extracted from the urine in pregnant women, tested in a lab for potency, and an assay is performed.

Medical Uses of HCG

Men

- HCG is a medication approved by the FDA for the medical treatment of Hypogonadism (very low testosterone) by stimulating the testes to produce more testosterone naturally. It naturally raises testosterone levels in men.

Women

- HCG therapy is used to treat infertility in high doses by stimulating ovulation and allows for the final maturation of eggs.

- During pregnancy if the mother does not eat enough to nourish the fetus, the hCG will help provide adequate nourishment by obtaining calories from the mother's fat reserves and feed the baby via the placenta.

Mechanism of hCG for Weight Loss

Men

- Elevated testosterone levels may result in an increase in metabolism

- The hCG hormone stimulates the hypothalamus in the brain to release abnormal fat reserves when on low calorie diet (below 800 calories)

- Spares lean muscle tissue

- The body may continue to burn more calories after the hCG therapy has been completed.

- Men achieve more weight loss than women due to their physiologic higher metabolic rate

Women

- Elevated hormone levels on small scale resulting in an increased metabolism

- The hCG hormone stimulates the hypothalamus in the brain to release abnormal fat reserves when on low calorie diet (below 800 calories)

- Spares lean muscle tissue

Average Weight Loss Results for Women in 6 Weeks

- Women who carefully follow the 800 Calorie hCG Diet Protocol may lose about **25-35** pounds in 40 days. Equivalent to ½- ¾ of a pound per day.

Contributing Factors:

* Women of child bearing age tend to lose more weight due to higher metabolic and hormone levels than menopausal women. Average loss may range from **30-35** pounds.

* Surgical hysterectomy, menopausal, and patients with thyroid disease may lose an average of **25** pounds in 40 days.

Average Weight Loss Results for Men in 6 Weeks

- Men who carefully follow the 800 Calorie hCG Diet Protocol may lose an average of **35-45** pounds in 40 days.

- About 1 pound per day

Contributing Factors:

* Men in general have a higher metabolic rate than women and more lean muscle mass

* A small increase in testosterone production may help raise the metabolic rate

Metabolic Action

- HCG is believed to cause the hypothalamus gland in the brain which regulates the thyroid, metabolic rate, adrenal glands, and storage of fat, to release and mobilize stored nutrients within the fat cells by shrinking and draining the fat cell's contents.

- The liquefied nutrients are then released into the bloodstream for the body to utilize as a source of natural energy.

- It is believed that up to 2,000 calories or more may be delivered in a single day, thus decreasing hunger, increasing energy and metabolism.

Most Commonly Asked Question

Would I lose the same amount of weight without taking HCG?

Answer - Most likely, Yes

However, restricting calories without the use of hCG may cause the following:

- Loss of precious lean muscle

- Decreased metabolism from muscle loss

- Increased hunger

- Increased irritability

- Increased fatigue and lack of energy

Chapter 3

Phase 1- (Pre-diet) Cleansing

This phase is recommended for dieters to follow for 2-4 weeks BEFORE starting the hCG diet treatment.

How to prepare your body for the hCG diet

• Start a 2-week Total Body Colon Cleanse to assist in deceasing the colon of toxins and waste that can slow down weight loss.

• Take a 15-day or 30-day Candida Yeast Cleanse before or after the hCG Treatment Therapy. Candida yeast build-up over time may prevent weight loss, depress the immune system, and slow down metabolism. The Candida cleanse should not be taken with the 2-week Total Body Cleanse. Take the Candida cleanse before the Total Body Cleanse or in Phases 3 or 4.

• A Multi Vitamin/Mineral supplement is suggested immediately when starting Phase 1. It provides superior essential nutrients to every organ in your body to sustain a low calorie diet. Recommended for lifetime use. Take a Coral Calcium supplement with your daily multi-vitamin/mineral. Please obtain approval from your physician on how much added calcium you can take daily.

• Take all medications prescribed to you by your personal physician. I strongly recommend you inform your personal physician before you start the hCG diet program or any weight loss program.

- Walk at least 30 minutes per day or begin your own light exercise regimen, such as swimming, biking, Pilates, or yoga.

- Get some sun. Studies show that sunshine exposure on your skin daily can increase your Vitamin D blood levels. Vitamin D deficiency may put you at risk for certain cancers. Ask your doctor about ordering the Vitamin D 25-hydroxy serum blood test.

- Drink a minimum of ½ a gallon of bottled or filtered water and/or unsweetened tea daily.

- Eat grapefruit (if not contraindicated due to a prescription medication you are taking). Grapefruit has been scientifically proven to release fat.

- Bragg Apple Cider Raw Unfiltered Vinegar can be used on your salad and marinated on your daily proteins (meat, breast of chicken and white fish) or to add flavor to your steamed vegetables. You may even use it as a cooking oil substitute. Apple Cider Vinegar stimulates metabolism and cleansing of the internal organs. It is also powerful in helping to release stored fat cells and has been proven to have properties similar to grapefruit in the release of fat. Found at most major supermarkets.

- Use a Natural Sweetener. I recommend Stevia as the preferred sweetener on the hCG diet. Both liquid and powder forms can be found at most major supermarkets and whole food stores. If you use powdered stevia, make sure it doesn't contain dextrose (inulin is OK). Please avoid artificial sweeteners such as Splenda, Truvia, Equal, and Sweet'N Low.

- Eating breakfast helps to increase your metabolism, burn fat, decrease appetite, and increase your morning blood sugar for energy throughout the day. If you skip breakfast, your body may potentially store fat and you are 450% more likely to gain weight.

- Eat 6 times per day. This helps to increase your metabolism and release excess fat reserves. Small meals are healthier than large ones.

- Eat a salad with lunch or dinner or in between meals as a snack. Eating a salad made with fresh vegetables helps to stimulate digestion and adds fiber, which helps to regulate blood sugar.

- Try to eat organically grown meat, fruits, and vegetables. Organic food does not contain preservatives, chemicals, flavor enhancers, herbicides, pesticides, growth hormones, or antibiotics. If organic food is not accessible, then look for chicken products in your local supermarket that do not contain antibiotics; fish products that are not farm raised and only wild caught, and wash all fruits and vegetables thoroughly.

- Add Fiber. Fiber will help relieve constipation, reduce appetite, improve digestion, improve metabolism, and cleanse the body of micro-toxins. A potent fiber supplement that contains soluble and insoluble fiber will help promote maximum digestive health.

- Eliminate carbonated beverages including diet drinks. They can block calcium absorption, may cause nutritional deficiencies and potentially slow down digestion.

- Avoid high fructose corn syrup. This is a man-made highly-processed sugar that is found in thousands of products in your grocery store. High fructose corn syrup can increase insulin levels which promotes fat storage and may lead to obesity.

- Avoid complex carbohydrates in Phases 1, 2, & 3 such as: bread, pasta, potatoes, rice, oatmeal, cereal, nuts, legumes, and granola bars.

- Avoid canned food.

- Avoid all sweets and dairy products.

- No MSG (Monosodium Glutamate).

- No Fast Food.

- No Fried Food.

Why you should do a Pre-Diet Total Body Colon Cleanse?

It is essential to use a Colon Cleanse prior to starting any weight loss plan. Most of the food we eat contains substances such as herbicides, pesticides, growth hormones, antibiotics, preservatives, flavor enhancers, and artificial flavors that we ingest regularly. Nature did not intend for us to consume these substances.

As food travels through our gastrointestinal (GI) tract, useful nutrients are absorbed and what is left over passes through our system, but if the bowels become clogged or saturated with toxins, or experience a buildup of plaque, then their ability to absorb nutrients is compromised. Therfore, potentially slowing down weight loss. Over time toxins can build up within the intestinal wall and can cause problems with digestion, constipation, fatigue, abdominal pain, bloating, and weight gain.

The 800 Calorie hCG Diet Protocol suggests to avoid consuming these potentially harmful substances in your daily diet, especially before and during the hCG Diet Phase 2 calorie restriction and hCG medication phase. Observing the nutritional content information and product label may be of some help. Additionally, it is important to use a Total Body Colon Cleanse which can also help rid the body of these toxins from the colon, kidney, liver, lungs, skin, bloodstream, and lymphatic system. This will help keep your GI tract running smoothly, restore the body to optimal health, improve the immune system, and promote healthy weight loss.

It is not recommended to start more than 1 colon cleanse at the same time.

Chapter 4

PHASE 2 - hCG DIET (Injections or Drops)

DAYS 1-2 (Loading Days)

- Weigh yourself right when you wake up, without clothing, after you have emptied your bladder. Record your weight on a weight loss tracking sheet.

How to Calculate Your hCG Diet Phase 2 Weight Loss

Day 1 170 **load**
Day 2 173 **load**
Day 3 175
Day 4 169
Day 5 167
Day 6 166
Day 7 165

'Loading weight' is not included as part of the dieter's "total weight loss". Loading weight is considered to be "artificial" or inflated weight gained and should not be included in the total weight lost. Weigh yourself on the morning of your first hCG medication day which is loading day 1 and weigh on the morning of loading day 2. Here is how to accurately chart your daily progress: By day 7, the dieter has lost 5 pounds, not 10.

*** There are many dieters that include loading weight as part of their total weight loss. Although I do not support this method, perhaps there is some degree of a psychological benefit which gives the dieter increased confidence to continue the challenges of weight loss.

- Take the hCG as directed on loading days 1 and 2

- Please eat fats and complex carbohydrates (starches) on Day 1 and 2 **ONLY**. These are your **LOAD** days. This will increase your body's fat stores to prepare you for the less than 800 calorie per day limit on days 3-40. This is the time to indulge with your favorite foods. Those who do not load may lose less weight.

- Drink a minimum of half your body's weight in ounces of bottled/filtered water or tea throughout the day. Do not drink tap water.

Loading Foods

Nuts – walnuts, macadamia, cashews, almonds

Fats/Oils - Mayo, avocados, coconut oil, butter, peanut butter

Dairy - Ice cream, heavy creams blended with fruit and drink it, half and half creamer, whole milk, whipping cream, whole eggs cooked in butter.

Starches w/ FAT - Pasta with heavy alfredo sauce, bread and butter, bagels with cream cheese and butter, potato skins or baked potato with cheddar cheese, sour cream, bacon and loads of butter, shredded beef chimi's with flour tortilla, bean burritos.

All Deep Fried Foods - onion rings, chili cheese French fries with sour cream.

Sweets - Turtle Cheesecake, peanut butter, e'clairs, donuts, cupcakes, pastries, candy bars, pies, cakes.

Meat - Greasy bacon cheeseburgers, rib eye steak, sausage, pork spare ribs, rump roast, bacon.

DAYS 3-40

Weigh yourself right when you wake up, without clothing, and after you have emptied your bladder. Record your weight on a weight loss tracking sheet.

- Take the hCG as directed.

- Drink ½ to a gallon of bottled or filtered water throughout the day.

- You must eat everything as described in Phase 2. Do not skip meals. Your total caloric intake will be between 550-800 calories per day, which consists of protein, vegetables, salad, and fruit. See the 800 calorie sample menu provided.

DAYS 41-43

- Stop taking the hCG. Continue to follow the Phase 2 diet on days 41-43 because the hCG hormone is still in your blood stream.

Nutritional Supplements

Importance of Vitamins and Minerals

What are vitamins and minerals? Vitamins and minerals are essential for the normal functioning of our bodies and are necessary for growth and vitality. Lack of them can lead to acute and chronic disease. They are found in food and supplements, but diet alone may not be enough. Particularly when you are on a weight-loss program, it is crucial that you receive adequate vitamins and minerals. People who are vitamin and mineral deficient may crave sweets, carbohydrates, and fat. When our bodies get the nutrition they need to function properly, we do not crave these things. Even if you eat six meals a day, you may still be deficient in nutrients your body needs. The food today is highly processed and the soil where most of our food is grown has been over utilized and is missing important nutrients needed to properly grow vitamin and mineral enriched foods. The vitamins and minerals we recommend are found to help ensure that while losing weight you are getting the proper nutrition to maintain optimal cellular health and diminish nutritional deficiencies. These deficiencies may cause cravings and addictions for the foods that may cause us to gain weight. These supplements are important to take before, during, and after a weight-loss program to maintain results and optimize health.

Recommended Supplements on P2 & P3

Multi-Vitamin/Mineral Whole Food Supplement

Whole Food Vitamins and Minerals are an essential part of any weight loss program. They help maintain and support adequate nutrients to the tissues, cells, and vital organs in the body. They also help in maintaining energy levels especially on a low calorie diet plan. Recommended vitamins include: A, B1, B2, B3, B5, B6, B12, C, D3, E, K1, Alpha Lipoic Acid,, Biotin, Calcium, Chromium, Copper, CoQ10, Folic Acid, Lutein, Magnesium, Manganese, Quercetin, Selenium and Zinc. Calcium and Vitamin D3 are essential in protecting muscle and bones.

Essential Fatty Acids - Omega 3, 6

There are only two Essential Fatty Acids: Alpha-linolenic acid (omega-3) and Linoleic acid (omega-6). The primary function of Essential Fatty Acids is to regulate the functioning of the body such as heart rate, blood pressure, blood clotting, fertility, and conception. They also assist with immune function by regulating inflammation and encouraging the body to fight infection. Essential Fatty Acids are the "good fats" that the body cannot synthesize and can only be obtained through diet. Essential fatty acids help support the cardiovascular, reproductive, and nervous systems which are needed while on a restricted calorie intake.

Fat Burner/Calcium pyruvate

Pyruvic acid is a natural substance already made in the human body. Higher levels of pyruvic acid in the bloodstream assist in calorie and fat burning and help speed up weight loss. Doctors recommend 1500-3000 mg with breakfast in the morning. This will help boost your metabolism for the entire day.

Candida Colon Cleanse

Candida albicans is yeast normally found in the digestive tract. This yeast can proliferate, upsetting the balance in the gastro-intestinal track, giving rise to problems such as rectal itching, diarrhea, constipation, bloating, skin problems, and many other issues. The goal of the Candida Cleanse is to decrease the amount of yeast to a normal and manageable level. This product is formulated with all-natural herbal and mineral ingredients used to support overgrowth of Candida yeast. Recommended for use before Phase 1 or in Phases 3 & 4.

Pre-Diet Phase 1 - Total Body Colon Cleanse

It is essential to use a Colon Cleanse prior to starting any weight loss plan. Most of the food that we eat contains flavor enhancers such as herbicides, pesticides, growth hormones, antibiotics, preservatives and artificial flavors that we ingest regularly. Nature did not intend for us to consume these substances. As food travels through our gastrointestinal tract, useful nutrients are absorbed, and what is left over passes through our system, but if the bowels become clogged or saturated with toxins, or experience a buildup of plaque, then their ability to absorb nutrients is compromised, therefore potentially slowing down weight loss. Over time, toxins can build up within the intestinal wall and can cause problems with digestion, constipation, fatigue, abdominal pain, bloating and weight gain.

PHASE 2 – hCG D!

Your Daily Intake at a Glance

Drink half your body's weight in ounces

2-3 fruit servings *

3 protein servings (egg whites are included as 1 protein)

2 green fiber-rich vegetable servings

1 small salad

Dieter's with Type 2 diabetes or insulin resistance should adjust accordingly

hCG Essentials

- Bragg Organic Apple Cider Vinegar
- Stevia Natural Sweetener
- All Natural Sea Salt or Pink Himalayan
- Garlic-Pepper Grinder • Food Scale
- George Foreman Grill
- Accurate Weight Scale • Tape Measure
- Hand-held fat-percentage monitor (optional)
- Pre-diet - Total Body Detox Cleanse (2 weeks)
- Whole Food Multi-Vitamin/Mineral, Vitamin D3, Calcium & Essential Fatty Acids

(Get approval from your doctor before taking a new supplement)

PHASE 2 - MENU

DRINK

Bottled or filtered water (no tap water)

Mineral water

Black coffee

Whole, skim, unsweetened Coconut or Almond or milk *Soy milk is not preferred but is allowed. (ONLY 2 tbsp/ day allowed)

Herbal Teas - Black, Green, Oolong, & Yerba Mate (no diet teas) Smooth Move as needed

NO alcoholic beverages

NO soda or diet soda, no diet drinks, no fruit or vegetables juices, no canned drinks

BREAKFAST

Drink plenty of tea and bottled or filtered water. You may have 1 fruit for breakfast and 3 egg whites.

LUNCH & DINNER

Lunch and dinner should be prepared with the same set of food choices: 1 protein, 1 fiber vegetable, 1 fruit, and 1 small salad with lunch. Eat your salad with lunch or as a snack. Avoid eating salad with dinner, as this meal should be lighter than your meal at lunch. The salad does not count as your fiber veggie serving, nor do the allowed 'toppers' or water veggies.

PROTEIN

Choose 1 of the following <u>proteins</u> for lunch and dinner. Proteins should be weighed raw (4 oz is 1 serving) then cooked.

*   **<u>Red Meat</u>**- Filet mignon (the leanest), top sirloin, T-bone, organic grass fed beef, buffalo, veal, NO TURKEY.

*   **<u>Chicken</u>**- Organic preferred or antibiotic free boneless breast of chicken (skinless), white meat only. Do not buy chicken that contains added rib meat, it may be loaded with sodium.

*   **<u>White Fish ONLY</u>**- Examples include: tilapia, cod, halibut, sea bass, sole, flounder, grouper, shrimp, lobster, scallops, oysters and crab. Any white fish is acceptable. No salmon….it is orange!

*   Grill or bake your proteins. Do not use any butter or margarine. Use organic cold pressed extra virgin olive oil or coconut oil in moderation. In order to use sparingly, place desired cooking oil in a separate spray bottle so there is just enough to coat your pan.

VEGETABLES (2 servings per day)

Choose 1 serving of **green** <u>vegetables</u> for lunch and dinner.

Portion: Eat 1 cup of cooked dark green fiber-rich vegetables (1.5 cups raw). These can be eaten steamed, grilled or raw. If it isn't green, do not eat it. Some exceptions are listed below. All vegetables must be fresh or fresh frozen. Canned vegetables are strictly prohibited.

What are the dark green fiber-rich vegetables?

Any dark green vegetable such as asparagus, spinach, broccoli, green beans, green bell pepper, cabbage etc..(see list below).You are required to eat 1 cup serving of cooked dark green fiber-rich veggies for lunch and for dinner. Veggies have been proven to increase digestion and assist with weight loss. They are also loaded with essential vitamins and minerals. Please do NOT substitute a tomato or cucumber as your veggie serving. These are "water vegies" and are not dark green fiber rich vegetables.

Green fiber-rich vegetables -Two servings daily

DO NOT mix green fiber-rich veggies on this list. **Portions:** 1 cup cooked or 1.5 cups raw served with lunch and dinner.

Asparagus	Green beans
Artichokes	Green bell peppers
Broccoli	Green zucchini
Brussels sprouts	Jalapeno
Cabbage	Leek
Collard greens	Spinach

NO peas	**NO** lima beans
NO cauliflower	**NO** soy beans
NO mushrooms	

Phase 2 'Water Veggies'
(for protein marinades or to mix in salad)

Celery	Red onion
Chard	White onion
Chicory	Green leaf lettuce
Cucumber	Red radish
Fennel	Daikon radish
Green onion	Red tomato

You may mix 'water veggies' with your small lunch salad from the above list. They are the ONLY veggies that can be mixed together. You can also add them to marinades. For example, you can make Sonia's hCG Salsa which can be topped on a boneless breast of chicken or added to your scrambled 3 egg whites for breakfast. Be sure to include the calories of all water veggies consumed in your daily caloric total. Green pepper and jalapeno are not water veggies but may be included in your marinade salsa. These can be used for flavoring in small amounts as a topper for all your proteins including breakfast egg whites and you will not gain or stall. If you have been using other veggies not on this list and have steady losses, please continue your veggie program. What works for some may not work for others. The above veggies have all been tested in the clinical setting and are all approved for Phase 2.

SALAD (1 small per day)

You may eat a small side salad with your lunch or in between meals. Use any green leaf lettuce, tomato, fresh onion, red radishes, cucumber, and celery with Bragg-Organic Apple Cider Raw Unfiltered Vinegar or generic equivalent that contains NO FAT. Lemon juice may also be used as a salad dressing. Additional P2 approved salad dressings are listed in the recipes section is this book. You may mix the above 'water veggies' in your salad. Fat free/sugar free dressings with artificial sweeteners are not allowed.

FRUIT (2-3 per day - organic preferred)

Eat 2-3 fruits per day with your meals or in between. Reduce fruit servings accordingly if you are Type 2 diabetic or insulin resistant. Increase your protein and veggie serving sizes to compensate for the lost fruit calories in order to meet your daily caloric range.

1 whole grapefruit (med)

1 green or red apple (med)

1 handful of strawberries (6)

1 orange (med)

* There are no fruit substitutes*** (Juice from 1 lemon per day for cooking or in water is OK)

* Try not to eat the same protein, vegetable, or fruit twice in the same day if possible. Metabolic activity may increase by following this concept suggested by Dr. Simeons.

CONDIMENTS

- Bragg Organic Apple Cider Raw Unfiltered Vinegar or generic equivalent found at whole food and major grocery stores – (proven to release fat in your body)

- Sea Salt (sparingly)

- Apple Cider Vinegar - ACV has historically been known to be used for medicinal purposes and has claims that it assists as a fat burner. If you have no tolerance for apple cider vinegar, you can purchase capsules at most whole food stores. Take two capsules before each meal. Liquid ACV should never be taken without dilution. Mix it with your water so it doesn't burn as you swallow.

- Stevia Natural Sweetener- This can be found at most whole food stores. Stevia comes in powder packet form and also a liquid. (Truvia is prohibited) If you buy in powered form, make sure it contains inulin and not dcxtrosc. Some brands mix the powdered stevia with other forms of sugar.

- Basil

- Bay Leaf

- Black Pepper

- Cayenne Pepper

- Celery Powder

- Chili Powder

- Cilantro

- Cinnamon

- Fennel

- Fresh Garlic, powder, paste or cloves

- Ginger Root
- Lemon Pepper
- Mustard Powder
- Onion Powder
- Oregano
- Paprika
- Parsley
- Red Pepper
- Rosemary
- Thyme
- Turmeric

Phase 2 Allowable Foods that Help Reduce Water Retention:

Cabbage	Asparagus	Lettuce
Cucumbers	Brussels Sprouts	Tomatoes

Egg Allergy Breakfast Alternatives

You may substitute of one of the following protein choices for your egg whites if you have an allergy or sensitivity to eggs:

4 oz. of 0% (non-fat) plain Greek yogurt with 1 fruit serving

4 oz. of 4% low sodium cottage cheese (no non-fat or low fat) with 1 fruit serving

1 serving – whey protein isolate shake with one fruit serving

* There are many protein shakes on the market but very few which do not contain ingredients that should be avoided during P2.

Please note: Ideally, your protein shakes should be made from whey protein isolate only and should NOT contain any of the following ingredients:

Acesulfame potassium (Sunett, Sweet One)
Aspartame (Equal, NutraSweet)
Artificial flavors
Dyes / Artificial coloring
DATEM
Dextrose
Diglycerides & Monoglycerides
High fructose corn syrup
Maltodextrin
Malitol syrup
Modified food starch
Saccharin (Sugar Twin, Sweet'N Low)
Sucralose (Splenda)
Sodium Caseinate

- Note: The above suggested alternatives were not tested in the clinical setting and are experimental. Please discontinue use if you do not experience steady losses.

Phase 2 - < 800 calorie

(Sample menu)

	Calories	Protein	Carbs	Fat	Sodium
Breakfast *(1 protein, 1 fruit)*					
3 large egg whites	51.0	10.5	0.6	0.3	164.5
6 medium strawberries (1 cup)	57.5	1.2	13.5	0.7	1.5
Totals	**108.5**	**11.7**	**14.1**	**1.0**	**166.0**

Morning snack *(1 fruit)*	Calories	Protein	Carbs	Fat	Sodium
½ large or 1 small green apple	52.4	2.0	16.2	0.4	2.0
Totals	**52.4**	**2.0**	**16.2**	**0.4**	**2.0**

Lunch *(1 protein, 1 vegetable, 1 salad)*	Calories	Protein	Carbs	Fat	Sodium
4 oz. chicken breast cooked (no skin)	188.0	28.0	0.0	2.5	71.25
1 cup asparagus	40.0	6.0	7.0	1.0	3.0
Finely chop asparagus to measure 1 cup					
1 bowl small salad, 1 tsp. apple cider vinegar	44.0	1.4	11.8	0.0	0.2
Enjoy a salad with lunch, dinner or as a snack					
Totals	**272.0**	**35.4**	**18.8**	**3.5**	**74.45**

Afternoon snack (1 fruit)	Calories	Protein	Carbs	Fat	Sodium
1 small orange	45.0	0.9	11.3	0.1	0.0
Totals	45.0	0.9	11.3	0.1	0.0

Dinner (1 protein, 1 vegetable)	Calories	Protein	Carbs	Fat	Sodium
4 oz. flounder	130.0	26.0	9.0	1.8	111.0
1 cup broccoli cooked	45.0	5.0	9.0	0	29.0
Optional salad					
Totals	175	31.0	18	1.8	140
Grand Totals	652.90	81.00	78.4	6.8	82.45

*Prolonged use of a very low-fat diet may lead to essential fatty acid deficiency. Supplementation with a multi-vitamin/mineral is also recommended during this phase.

Phase 2 hCG Recipes

Phase 2 - Beverages

Frozen Cappuccino
1 cup crushed ice
5 drops of chocolate stevia
5 drops of Valencia orange
1 cup of black coffee
1 tbsp. of whole, skim, or unsweetened coconut or almond milk

Mix in blender until smooth. Pour into glass and serve!

Lemonade
6 lemons
1 stevia pkg.

Pour lemon juice into 8 oz. glass, add stevia, chill and serve!

Mint Green Tea
2 quarts of bottled or filtered water
5 green tea bags
5-6 packets of Stevia
4-5 mint leaves

Place warm to hot water into pitcher. Add green tea bags and mint leaves. Allow to steep overnight. Remove tea bags and mint leaves. Stir in Stevia. Great hot or cold.

Orange Julius

1 orange, peeled and sectioned
5-10 drops vanilla crème liquid Stevia
½ cup of ice add more if desired
Bottled or filtered water as needed

Place all ingredients in a blender and mix until smooth. Pour into a glass and serve.

Strawberry Chocolate Smoothie

6-7 frozen or fresh strawberries
1 cup crushed ice
1 T milk
10-15 drops of chocolate liquid Stevia

Place all ingredients in a blender and mix until smooth. Pour into a glass and serve.

Strawberry Lemonade

2 large mashed strawberries
Juice of ½ a lemon
8 oz. of bottled or filtered water
Ice desired amount
1 package of Stevia

Mix mashed strawberries and lemon juice in a glass. Add bottled or filtered water and mix well. Pour over Ice and add Stevia and stir.

Sweet and Sour Lemonade
2 quarts of bottled or filtered water
2 lemons
4 packets of Stevia
Lemon slices for garnish
Ice cubes

Place water into a pitcher. Add juice only from two lemons and Stevia and stir. Add desired amount of ice and garnish with lemon slices.

V-8 Tomato Juice
*May also be used as a marinade for meats.
3 large tomatoes
1 tsp. cilantro
½ tsp. Stevia
½ tsp. garlic paste
¼ tsp. cumin
1/8 tsp. celery seed
Juice from ½ a lemon
Pinch of sea salt and ground black pepper

Combine all ingredients in a blender and puree until desired consistency. Place in refrigerator until chilled or serve over ice.

Phase 2 - Soups & Salads

Beef & Cabbage Soup

4 oz. sirloin beef thinly sliced
1 cup of cabbage chopped
3 garlic cloves minced
2 cups of bottled or filtered water
¼ tsp. cumin
¼ tsp. cayenne pepper
Pinch of sea salt and ground black pepper to desired taste

Heat a saucepan using medium heat. When hot, add 1 cup water. Bring water to a boil and then add the beef and garlic. By the time the water has boiled off the beef should be cooked, if not add water as needed. When the water has boiled off you should see the "browning" on the pan from the beef. Add bottled or filtered water. This will create a rich broth. Add chopped cabbage and remaining ingredients until the cabbage is cooked to desired consistency.

Broth
* Broth is an ingredient in many recipes and can be stored in the freezer*

4 oz. boneless chicken breast
1 tsp. parsley
1 tsp. onion powder
1 tsp. minced garlic
1 tsp. thyme
1tsp rosemary
1 tsp. oregano
1 tsp. basil
1 bay leaf
½ tsp. sea salt
½ tsp. ground pepper
Bottled or filtered water

Fill sauce pan ¾ full of bottled or filtered water. Bring to a boil. Add all ingredients and boil for 20 minutes. Remove boiled chicken and save for a meal. Strain out bay leaf and seasonings. Let broth cool. Skim off any fat from surface. Serve and Refrigerate unused portions.

Green Onion Soup
Green onions as desired
2 cups of bottled or filtered water
1 tsp. parsley
½ tsp. paprika
½ tsp. sea salt
½ tsp. dill
½ tsp. thyme
1/8 tsp. cayenne pepper
1/8 tsp. celery seed

Briefly steam green onions until tender. Preheat sauce pan over medium heat. Chop green onions and sauté in sauce pan with remaining ingredients EXCEPT water. Add bottled or filtered water and simmer for 30 minutes and serve.

Spicy Chicken Soup

4 oz. chicken breast
½ cup tomatoes, diced
1 jalapeno pepper- *add three punctures with a knife to release flavors*
2 T cilantro
2 tsp. garlic powder
1 green onion
½ T apple cider vinegar
1 tsp. lemon juice
6 drops lemon Stevia
1 cup broth *(refer to recipe)*
1 cup of bottled or filtered water

In a small pot, add broth, bottled or filtered water, chicken, jalapeno and garlic powder. Remove jalapeno pepper after about 5 minutes or to desired flavor of jalapeno. Cook chicken through and remove from broth, let cool and shred with fingers. Put tomatoes, cilantro, and a 1-3 inch piece of the pepper in blender. Pulse until creamy. Add puree to broth and simmer a few minutes over medium heat. Lower heat to medium-low; add chicken, green onion, lemon juice, Stevia and apple cider vinegar. Simmer 15 minutes. Top with fresh green onion and cilantro.

Protein Salad
4 oz. of any protein desired
1 cup lettuce, shredded
4 cherry tomatoes cut in halves
1 T lemon juice
Sea salt and ground black pepper for desired taste
Desired spices

Combine all ingredients and mix well and serve.

Apple Chicken Salad
4 oz. grilled chicken breast
4 celery stalks, diced
4 T lemon juice
1 green apple, diced
1 package of Stevia
Pinch of cinnamon

Combine all ingredients and mix thoroughly and serve.

Cucumber Salad
1 cucumber peeled and sliced thinly
1 tsp. apple cider vinegar
1 tsp. dill
½ tsp. Stevia
1 T cilantro, chopped
Ground black pepper & sea salt

Combine all ingredients EXCEPT cucumber and mix well. Toss in cucumbers. Cover and refrigerate. This tastes best if you wait at least one hour to before serving.

Phase 2 - Snacks

Applesauce

2 green apples, peeled and sliced thinly
1 package of Stevia
Cinnamon
¼ cup of bottled or filtered water

In a small sauce pan add apple slices. Sprinkle desired amount of cinnamon on to apples. Add bottled or filtered water and simmer on low heat. Cook to your desired texture. The firmer slices are the harder they are to mash. Firmer slices simulate apple pie filling. Add Stevia when apples are to your desired likeness. Makes 2 servings.

Cinnamon Grapefruit

Grapefruit cut into 2 halves
Cinnamon
1 package of Stevia

Preheat oven to broil. Take a knife around the inside peel of the grapefruit so that it cuts out the grapefruit from the peel. Keep peel in solid form and set aside. Separate the sections and place in a bowl. Sprinkle with cinnamon and Stevia. Place grapefruit back into peel. Place peels on cookie sheet and broil for 5 minutes or until caramelized.

Sautéed Garlic and Greens

6 garlic cloves
5 bunches of Swiss chard greens
1 squeeze of lemon
½ tsp. sea salt

Heat garlic in a large skillet over medium to low heat in a non-stick pan until garlic begins to turn golden. Transfer to a small bowl and set aside. Place greens and salt in skillet. Using tongs, turn greens until wilted enough to fit in pan. Cover pan. Cook 7-10 minutes occasionally tossing. Transfer greens to a colander and drain. Return greens to pan and toss with reserved garlic. Squeeze with lemon before serving. Refrigerate left over greens in an air tight container for up to 3 days.

Steamed Cabbage

1 ½ cups cabbage
Juice from half a lemon
½ tsp. Dijon mustard *(refer to recipe)*
Pinch of sea salt and ground black pepper for desired taste

Place cabbage in a steamer. Cover and steam for 5-10 minutes until slightly tender. In a small mixing bowl, combine Dijon mustard and lemon juice. Place cabbage in bowl, add lemon and mustard mix and toss. Add sea salt and ground black pepper and serve.

Strawberries and Cream Sorbet
6-7 Strawberries
½ cup of Ice
7-10 drops of Vanilla Crème liquid Stevia *(add more for desired flavor)*

Pour all ingredients in a blender. Blend on high. Eat or freeze.

Veggies & Salsa
1-2 cups of allowed veggies
¼ cup of salsa *(refer to recipe)*

Cut up 1-2 cups of allowed veggies and dip in salsa.

Zesty Asparagus
2 cups asparagus, cleaned and woody end removed
¾ cup bottled or filtered water
½ T ginger root, minced
3 garlic clove, minced
lemon zest
Sea salt and ground black pepper for desired taste

Preheat pan over medium heat. Snap asparagus spears into 2-3 pieces. Add garlic and ginger to the pan and cook for 2-3 minutes. Add asparagus and bottled or filtered water. Bring to a boil for 5 minutes. Remove asparagus and top with lemon zest and pepper.

Phase 2 – Chicken Dishes

Crock-Pot Chicken
6 boneless skinless chicken breasts
4 onions cut into 1 inch pieces
1 bunch celery cut into 1 inch pieces
1 head garlic separated and peeled
2-3 cups water
Allowable spices

In crock-pot, layer 1/2 celery, 1/2 onion, garlic pieces and chicken breasts. Sprinkle chicken with a layer of spices. Top with remaining celery and onion and another layer of spices. Add water almost to top. Cook on low for 8-9 hours. Weigh chicken and enjoy!

Tai Chicken Wrap
1 extra-large iceberg lettuce leaf
4 oz. boneless skinless chicken breast
1/4 cup white onions, diced
1/4 cup green peppers, diced
3 cherry tomatoes, diced
pinch of black pepper
pinch of sea salt

Chop chicken breast into small square pieces. Cook chicken, onions and green peppers in pan. Place on top of lettuce leaf. Add diced tomatoes and season with black pepper and sea salt. Fold leaf lettuce in half and serve!

Chicken Broth

4 oz. chicken
Pinch of:
parsley
onion powder
garlic
thyme
rosemary
oregano
basil
bay leaf
sea salt
black pepper

Fill saucepan 3/4 full with water. Bring to boil. Add chicken and seasonings. Boil for 20 min. Remove boiled chicken and save for later. Strain out bay leaf & seasonings. Serve!

Chicken & Asparagus

4 oz. boncless skinless chicken breast
1 ½ cup asparagus, chopped
2 T onion, chopped
1 tsp. onion powder
1 minced garlic clove
Sea salt and ground black pepper for desired taste

Preheat oven to 375 degrees. Coat baking dish with organic olive oil cooking spray. Mix all ingredients together and pour into a small baking dish. Bake for 30 minutes or until bubbly and hot.

Chicken & Cabbage

4 oz. boneless skinless chicken breast
2 cups cabbage, shredded
1 tsp. Dijon mustard *(refer to recipe)*
¼ tsp. garlic powder
¼ cup of bottled or filtered water
Sea salt and ground pepper for desired taste

Slice chicken into bite sized pieces, Heat medium skillet on medium to high heat. Cook chicken for 2 minutes and add a bottled or filtered water to loose from bottom of pan. Turn and immediately add the cabbage. Stir frequently until cabbage starts to wilt and chicken is cooked through. Add mustard, garlic powder, salt and pepper. Pour into a serving dish.

Chicken Fajitas

4 oz. boneless skinless chicken breasts cut into strips
1 tsp. sea salt
½ tsp. ground black pepper
½ tsp. cumin
½ tsp. chili powder
½ tsp. onion powder
¼ tsp. garlic powder
¼ cup of bottled or filtered water
1 green pepper cut into strips
1 medium onion thinly sliced
2 T lime juice

In a zip-lock plastic bag combine the chili powder, salt, cumin, onion powder, garlic powder, and bottled or filtered water. Add chicken, bell pepper and onion. Seal and knead gently to coat. Refrigerate for 15 minutes. Heat a large nonstick skillet on medium heat Empty contents of bag into the skillet and cook stirring occasionally until vegetables are crisp and tender and chicken is cooked through. Remove from heat. Serve.

Chicken & Green Onions

4 oz. boneless skinless chicken breasts grilled and cubed
1 cup green onions, chopped
1 tsp. mustard powder
1 tsp. apple cider vinegar
¼ cup of bottled or filtered water
¼ tsp. garlic powder
Sea salt and ground pepper to taste

Coat a medium sized skillet with organic olive oil cooking spray. Preheat skillet over medium heat. Add green onions to skillet and stir fry until they begin to soften, approximately 2 minutes. Add chicken to skillet. Add bottled or filtered water and seasonings to taste. Stir and let cook 1-2 minutes or until chicken is warmed through and sauce is beginning to thicken. Serve.

Chicken in Tomato Sauce

4 oz. of boneless skinless grilled chicken breasts
1 medium size tomato
1 garlic clove minced
¼ tsp. onion powder
¼ tsp. oregano
¼ tsp. basil
¼ tsp. thyme

Slice up tomato and put in a sauce pan and sauté over medium heat for 5 minutes. While being heated occasionally, smash tomato with a spoon to soften. When your tomato is heated and softened it should have the consistency of thick spaghetti sauce. Add in chicken and spices and mix. Serve

Chicken Oregano
4 oz. boneless skinless chicken breast
1 ½ tsp. oregano
½ tsp. basil
½ cup broth *(refer to recipe)*
¼ garlic powder
¼ onion powder
Sea salt and ground black pepper for desired taste

Preheat oven to 350 degrees. Coat a small sized baking dish with organic olive oil cooking spray. Baste chicken in broth. Mix all spices together and coat chicken. Layer chicken in baking dish. Pour remaining broth in dish. Bake for 20 minutes or until chicken is cooked thoroughly.

Chicken Shish Kabobs
4 oz. boneless skinless chicken breasts cut into cubes
2 skewers
6 cherry tomatoes
1 small onion, cut in chunks
½ green pepper, cut in chunks
1 t lemon juice
Any allowed seasoning as desired

Arrange chicken and vegetables on skewers. Baste with lemon juice. Add desired seasonings and grill.

Citrus Chicken

4 oz. boneless skinless chicken breast
3 tomatoes, chopped
2 large leafs of lettuce
1 orange, peeled and cut into pieces
½ squeezed lemon
1 T basil
½ tsp. thyme
Sea salt and ground pepper for desired taste

Coat a medium sized skillet with organic olive oil cooking spray. Over medium heat, add chicken and coat with salt and pepper and squeeze lemon juice over chicken. Cook 4-5 minutes. Add chopped tomatoes, orange, basil and thyme. Simmer on low until chicken is cooked thoroughly. Serve on a bed of lettuce.

Phase 2 – Seafood

Curry Shrimp
4 oz. shrimp (peeled and deveined)
1/2 white onion, diced
3 garlic cloves, minced
1/8 cup distilled water
1/2 tsp. curry powder
1/4 tsp. cumin
•pinch of sea salt
•pinch of black pepper

Preheat pan over MED heat. Add onion and garlic. Cook for 8-10 minutes. Add shrimp, seasonings, and water. Mix & stir fry until cooked thoroughly and serve!

Garlic Shrimp
4 oz. shrimp (peeled & deveined)
4 garlic cloves, minced
1/2 cup hCG chicken broth
pinch black pepper
1/2 tsp. parsley
1/8 tsp. dried thyme
1/8 tsp. crushed dried red pepper
1 bay leaf

Heat non-stick pan over med heat. Mix ¼ cup broth with red pepper, minced garlic, and bay leaf. Add to pan. Cook less than a minute. Be sure not to burn the garlic. Add shrimp. Cook 3 minutes. Remove shrimp from pan Add the remainder of the 1/4 cup broth, parsley, & thyme. Bring to a boil. Cook for 1-2 min. until reduced by half. Return shrimp to pan & toss to coat. Discard bay leaf & serve!

Citrus Tilapia

4 oz. tilapia
1 tsp. dill
1 T lemon juice
1 T lime juice
1 minced garlic clove
¼ tsp. ground black pepper
¼ tsp. sea salt

Combine all ingredients EXCEPT tilapia in a dish and mix well. Coat tilapia in mixture and let marinate for 15-30 minutes. Coat a medium sized skillet with organic olive oil cooking spray. Heat over medium to low heat and cook tilapia 4 minutes per side or until fully cooked. Serve

Herbed Fish & Broccoli

4 oz. of any allowed white fish
4 oz. of broccoli, chopped
1 tomato, peeled and cut into small size pieces
¼ tsp. basil
¼ tsp. thyme
¼ tsp. oregano
3 T bottled or filtered water
Sea salt and ground black pepper for desired taste

Add all spices into the bottom of a medium sized skillet. Add fish on top and drizzle with lemon. Add broccoli and tomato with bottled or filtered water and cook over medium to low heat until fish is thoroughly cooked. Pour juices over fish and serve.

Lemon Pepper Fish & Asparagus

4 oz. of any allowed white fish
Non-stick aluminum foil
6-8 asparagus spears, wood ends removed
Juice of one lemon
1tsp. oregano
¼ tsp. sea salt
¼ tsp. ground black pepper

Preheat oven to 400 degrees. Tear off a large sheet of non-stick aluminum foil. In center of sheet, place asparagus spears and sprinkle with sea salt and ground black pepper. Place white fish on top of asparagus. In small mixing bowl combine lemon juice and oregano and pour over fish. Fold up edges and completely seal on all sides. Bake 10-20 minutes or until fish becomes flaky. Serve.

Lobster in Tomato Sauce

4 oz. raw lobster tail cut in slices
4 oz. organic no sugar added tomato paste
2 tomatoes, chopped
3 T lemon juice
1 minced clove of garlic
1 T onion powder
1 bay leaf
2 T bottled or filtered water
¼ tsp. thyme
¼ tsp. parsley
Pinch of cayenne pepper
Sea salt and ground black pepper to taste

In a medium skillet, sauté lobster in lemon juice and bottled or filtered water. Add onion powder, garlic, tomatoes, tomato paste and spices. Simmer for 15 minutes and serve.

Poached Halibut

4 oz. halibut
½ cup broth *(refer to recipe)*
2 T lemon juice
1 T onion, chopped
1 minced garlic clove
½ tsp. ginger
¼ tsp. lemon zest
¼ tsp. sea salt
¼ tsp. ground black pepper
Pinch of Stevia

Heat up broth in a small skillet. Add onion, lemon juice, garlic and spices. Add halibut to skillet. Poach halibut for 7-10 minutes until it is tender and fully cooked. Serve.

Phase 2 - Beef

Hamburger
4 oz. grass fed or lean ground beef
large lettuce leaf
tomato slice
grilled or raw white onion
hCG dijon mustard

Place beef patty in center of lettuce leaf, add toppings and serve!

Baked Steak & Tomatoes
4 oz. sirloin steak
2 cups tomato, diced
3 minced garlic cloves
2 tsp. oregano
2 tsp. basil
¼ tsp. chili powder
¼ tsp. ground black pepper

Preheat oven to 350 degrees. Place 1 cup of diced tomatoes in a casserole dish. Add steak on top of tomatoes and top with minced garlic. In a mixing bowl, combine 1 cup tomatoes, oregano, basil, ground black pepper and chili powder. Place mixture on top of steak. Cover dish with aluminum foil and bake for 50 minutes.

Beef & Ginger
4 oz. of sirloin beef cut into thin strips
¼ broth *(refer to recipe)*
1 T apple cider vinegar
3 T lemon juice
3 T green onions, chopped
¼ tsp. grated ginger
3 T bottled or filtered water
2 minced garlic cloves
Sea salt and ground black pepper for desired taste
Pinch of Stevia

In medium skillet, sauté spices, ginger and all liquid ingredients. Add beef and stir fry gently. Periodically de-glaze pan by adding small amounts of bottled or filtered water. Add green onions and serve.

Beef Lettuce Wraps
4 oz. of organic grass fed beef
2 T taco seasoning *(refer to recipe)*
2 large lettuce lcaves
¼ cup green pepper, chopped
¼ onion, chopped
3 T salsa *(refer to recipe)*

In medium skillet, brown the beef with taco seasoning. Half way through cooking, add in green peppers and onion and continue to sauté until beef is fully cooked. Let cool a few minutes. Scoop beef mixture on to lettuce leaves. Top with salsa and wrap up leaves. Serve.

Beef Roll-ups

4 oz. of organic grass feed beef
1 cup of broth *(refer to recipe)*
2 T onion, chopped
2 large cabbage leaves slightly steamed
1 minced garlic clove
¼ tsp. garlic powder
¼ tsp. onion powder

Preheat oven to 375 degrees. In a medium skillet combine beef, garlic, onion, and spices and cook until brown. Spoon beef mixture on to the cabbage leaves. Tuck in ends and roll up like a burrito. Place rolls in a baking dish and pour broth on bottom of dish. Brush cabbage with broth for moisture. Bake for 30 minutes and periodically spoon sauce over cabbage to keep moist.

Pot Roast

4 oz. sirloin steak
1 tsp. onion powder
1 tsp. garlic powder
1 ½ cup of broth *(refer to recipe)*
½ tsp. thyme
½ tsp. basil
¼ tsp. sea salt
¼ tsp. ground black pepper

Mix all ingredients EXCEPT steak in a mixing bowl. Place steak in a crock pot. Pour mixture over steak. Cook on low for several hours until steak is cooked as desired.

Phase 2 - Condiments

Strawberry Vinaigrette Dressing
6-8 fresh frozen strawberries
2 oz. apple cider vinegar
1 stevia packet

Place 6-8 fresh frozen strawberries in a bowl. Sprinkle Stevia on top of frozen strawberries and allow to defrost. Pour strawberry juice into separate bowl and add apple cider vinegar. Add pulp from defrosted strawberries if desired, mix and serve!

Deli Mustard
1/4 cup mustard powder or seed
1/8 cup apple cider vinegar
pinch of sea salt
1/8 cup distilled water
add allowed spices as desired

Dijon Mustard
1/4 mustard powder or seed
1/8 apple cider vinegar
pinch of sea salt
pinch of turmeric
pinch of fennel
1/8 distilled water
1 pkg. stevia

Sonia's hCG Salsa
4 large tomatoes, diced
1 large white onion, diced
1 lemon (juice only)
1/4 green bell pepper, diced
1/4 garlic clove (minced)
1/2 cup finely chopped cilantro
1 tsp. apple cider vinegar
sea salt (2 pinches)
black pepper (2 pinches)

Mix and chill for 3 hours and enjoy!

Asian Marinade
15-20 drops English Toffee Stevia
1 ½ cups of bottled or filtered water
½ tsp. ground ginger
¼ tsp. garlic powder
¼ tsp. ground black pepper

Combine all 5 ingredients and mix well. Marinate on choice of meat.

Cajun Seasoning
1 T chili powder (no salt)
1 T paprika
1 tsp. garlic powder
1 tsp. onion powder
½ tsp. oregano
½ tsp. thyme
½ tsp. cayenne pepper
½ tsp. ground black pepper
¼ tsp. sea salt

Combine ingredients and store in air-tight container or plastic sealed bag. Rub on fish or meats before cooking.

Citrus Salad Dressing
1 T lemon juice
1 packet of Stevia
¼ tsp. ground black pepper
¼ tsp. sea salt

Combine all 5 ingredients and mix well. Add on salad, shrimp or vegetables.

Cocktail Sauce
¼ cup of Ketchup *(refer to hCG ketchup recipe)*
1 T Lemon Juice
Sea Salt and black pepper optional for taste

Mix ingredients together. Add more sea salt and black pepper for desired taste.

hCG Ketchup
1 can of organic no sugar added tomato paste
2 T onion powder
½ tsp. sea salt
½ tsp. vinegar
1 tsp. paprika
1/8 tsp. cinnamon
2 packets of stevia

Mix all ingredients thoroughly in a medium sized mixing bowl. Store in a plastic squeeze bottle and refrigerate.

Meat Marinade
2 cloves garlic, minced
2 tsp. lemon pepper
2tsps. lemon juice
2 tsp. ground black pepper

Combine all ingredients and marinate on choice of meat.

Another Meat Marinade
2 T paprika
1 T stevia
1 T cumin
1 T ground black pepper
1 T chili powder
1 T sea salt

Combine ingredients and store in air-tight container or plastic sealed bag. Rub on meats before cooking.

Taco Seasoning
1 T chili Powder
2 tsp. onion powder
1 tsp. cumin
1 tsp. garlic powder
1 tsp. ground pepper
1 tsp. paprika
1 tsp. oregano
1 tsp. sea salt

Combine ingredients and store in air-tight container or plastic sealed bag. Great to use when cooking organic grass feed beef or extra lean ground beef.

For a comprehensive Cookbook, get your copy of **The Best Diet's Ultimate hCG Recipe Cookbook** (over 156 Phase 2 & Phase 3 recipes, includes food preparation, grocery shopping & check-off lists, food journaling tips and many helpful hCG dieting tips).

Available at www.hcgdoctorsgroup.com, Amazon, Barnes and Noble, and Borders online bookstores.

Phase 2: What is a Stall?

A weight loss stall while on phase 2 of the hCG diet can occur even when you have followed the diet strictly and have been perfect on protocol days before. You rush to the scale in the morning, so excited to see how much weight you have lost... and to your surprise, the scale has not moved. Everyone will experience their first stall somewhere between day 8 and day 11.

Why does a stall occur when you have been so strict and staying on protocol? After the first week on Phase 2, it is common for the body to fight you in dropping more weight. Your body is catching up with the rapid weight loss from the first 7-10 days which is where you will lose the most weight. Ignore this stall and move forward by staying POP (perfect on protocol) and the losses will come. They always do. Keep in mind that what you don't see on the scale, you are losing in inches, so it is best to keep accurate recorded measurements at least every 3 days.

Stalls can last anywhere from 1 day up to 5 days of no weight loss. A stall beyond 5 days is usually an indicator of another issue such as excess salt intake resulting in water retention, constipation, lactose intolerance that may cause intestinal inflammation and bloating, menses, illness, prescription medications, or eating off protocol.

The challenges of losing weight can definitely be frustrating at times. We all go through the highs and lows and try to accept what we see on the scale, even if it appears to be not in our favor. A stall is expected and is part of the program. Also, it is very important to remain positive about your weight loss. Studies have shown that dieters who maintain a positive attitude about their weight loss

ε more weight. Dieters that have a good
ɔort system will also lose more weight and
.ιr weight loss goals.

A weight loss stall is expected, so keep your chin up, move
onward, then downward on the scale.

Phase 2 - Stall Breakers

The following tips and techniques have been very effective
"stall breakers" during Phase 2 of the hCG protocol, though
some are also effective as a "correction" in Phase 3.

• Sonia's Cantaloupe Plateau Breaker

At bedtime, eat half of a medium sized cantaloupe (make
sure to cut it yourself) and drink 16 ounces of water right
before you lie down to sleep. You should lose between
0.5-3 pounds the following morning. Eating cantaloupe
assists in pulling water out of the fat cells and this action
works best while you are asleep. For dieters on the 500
calorie protocol, the 1/2 cantaloupe at bedtime will be your
second fruit of the day. For dieters on the 800 calorie
protocol, the 1/2 cantaloupe at bedtime will be your third
fruit of the day.

• Non-Fat 0% Fage Greek Yogurt Day
by Sonia Russell and Candice Ekberg

We have researched and tested the non-fat 0% Fage Greek
Yogurt as a stall breaker in phase 2. Full fat or 2 % is not
suggested. Although many dieters will drop pounds the
following day, we have observed the weight often creeps
back on over the next consecutive days if the full fat or 2%
has been used. This has not occurred when using non-fat

0 percent yogurt, and may be primarily due to the very high fat content in the full fat version. Dieters have reported excellent results with the 0% non- fat version. Suggested brands include: Fage, All Natural Brown Cow, and Dannon Oikos. We do suggest you still check your labels for high protein, low carb/sugar (dairy sugar only, no added) and zero fat. * PLAIN ONLY 0% NON-FAT GREEK YOGURT. Instructions: Buy #1 16 oz. tub of approved 0% NON FAT PLAIN Greek Yogurt, divide into 4 oz. servings and add 2 oz. of fresh berries per serving (strawberries or raspberries). Eat the 4 servings throughout the day. Continue drinking your regular daily fluids. *Depending on the brand chosen, please ensure your total caloric intake is above 500 calories. If not, add 1 extra oz. per serving of yogurt.

• Dr. Simeons Apple Day

Reduce your fluid intake by 1 quart and eat 6 apples throughout the day. This method typically eliminates excess fluids in the body and most dieters will lose about 2 pounds. This method is not recommended to be followed on a regular basis or for those with Type 2 diabetes.

• Dr. Simeons Steak Day

Drink as much fluid as possible throughout the day and then enjoy a large steak for dinner. You may have 1 tomato or an apple with your steak. Many dieters have reported a weight loss of about 2 pounds the following day.

Note: Atkins-based Fat Fast - NOT RECOMMENDED. We have seen too many people experience rebound gains after attempting this method as a stall breaker. Furthermore, it is actually dangerous for anyone with gall bladder issues to attempt.

• **Calcium pyruvate** has been touted by many medical professionals as one of the best natural fat burning supplements. Pyruvic acid is a natural substance already made in the human body. Higher levels of pyruvic acid in the bloodstream assist in calorie and fat burning and help to boost metabolism for the entire day. Note: for every 750mg of Calcium pyruvate, 125mg is actual calcium. The remainder is Pyruvic acid. Make sure to contact your personal physician before beginning a new supplement.

• Ask your prescribing hCG diet weight loss physician to increase your hCG dosage by 25 IU's daily until you lose weight and then resume the original dosage once the plateau has been broken. Do not attempt to increase your hCG dosage without the permission of your prescribing doctor.

• Drink Oolong, Black, and Green Tea, as they are made from the Camellia sinensius plant. There are only 3 types of tea that have significant health benefits - black, green, and oolong, all which increase metabolism and burn fat.

• Get enough sleep. Many dieters have reported that not enough sleep has reflected little or no weight loss on the following day. The reason this occurs is if you do not get at least 7 hours of sleep each night, especially on phase 3 when the body is stabilizing your metabolic rate, the body will increase the production of the hormone Ghrelin. Ghrelin also increases appetite and slows down metabolism resulting in the storage of fat.

• Intense exercise is not needed for success on the hCG diet. If you are on the 500 calorie protocol and have been lifting weights, consider limiting your physical activity to just walking on a treadmill for 30 minutes a day, as tolerated. Resistance training builds lean muscle mass.

Lean muscle weight may skew your weight loss (scale. Dieters following the 800 calorie hCG diet pr may participate in more exercise to include some ⎯ᴚ⎯ resistance training or 30 minutes of low impact aerobic activity, only as tolerated. However, it is best to wait until you have finished the Phase 2 hCG therapy.

• Increase your fluid intake. As a rule of thumb, make sure you are drinking half your body weight in ounces per day. Additional fluids will assist in promoting adequate digestion, help prevent constipation and may help to flush out toxins and fat. If you are not drinking enough water daily, your body will store water as a means of protection.

• Try increasing your protein by half an ounce. You may not be eating enough calories per day. Avoid consuming less than 500 calories daily because your body may store fat and other nutrients or you may not lose any weight. In some cases you may actually gain.

• Limit eating red meat to only 1 or 2 times per week. Red meat digests slowly in the bowel and may slow down weight loss. Avoid eating red meat at dinner time.

• Make sure you are not using garlic salt or salt substitutes. Garlic powder and sea salt are acceptable. Products such as Mrs. Dash and No Salt are not approved.

• Do not mix green vegetables. For example, do not mix asparagus and cabbage together. However, you can mix veggies in your salad such as lettuce, tomato, and onion (these are mainly made of water). Just remember that green fiber vegetables should not be mixed.

• Discontinue Grissini bread sticks, Melba toast, and Wasa crackers. These are not allowed on the 800 Calorie Protocol.

• Do not eat the same protein, vegetable, or fruit more than once in the same day. For example, do not eat tilapia for lunch and dinner or half a grapefruit for breakfast and the other half for lunch. Metabolism increases when the body has different foods to break down and digest.

• Make sure there are no antibiotics, flavor enhancers, or added rib meat in your chicken or other protein sources.

• Do not eat any canned food products. Many canned food products contain high fructose corn syrup, preservatives, elevated sodium and flavor enhancers that may slow down weight loss.

• Make sure you buy your proteins raw and without any marinades. Most store bought marinades contain high levels of sugar or sodium.

• For women, your menstrual cycle may cause a water weight gain of 2-5 pounds. Be aware of the date of your last menstrual cycle and never begin the hCG diet right when you start your period.

• Discontinue the use of Braggs Aminos, as it is LOADED with sodium.

• If you are not having regular bowel movements, a fiber supplement such as over the counter Senna is recommended by doctors to be taken daily. It is possible to hold 5 or more pounds of stool in the colon. High protein low fat diets most often will cause constipation. If you have not had a bowel movement for 5 days, an over the counter laxative suppository should be taken. If you do not experience relief then please contact your doctor's office for further instruction.

• Raw Unfiltered Organic Apple Cider Vinegar is the star condiment on the 800 Calorie Protocol. If you suffer from acid reflux or just dislike the taste, consider taking Apple Cider Vinegar Capsules found at most health food stores. ACV has been scientifically proven to release fat within the body and contains similar properties that have been found in grapefruit.

Chapter 5

800 Calorie Protocol Facts & Tips

The Importance of Drinking Water

It is important to understand how essential water is in order to reach your weight loss goals while on the hCG diet plan or any weight loss program. In fact, this remains true for anyone, whether you want to lose weight, gain weight or maintain your current weight! It is a well-known fact that we all should be following the "8 x 8 rule" which is drinking eight (8-ounce) glasses of water a day in order for our bodies to maintain optimal function. We all know we cannot survive without water, but just why is it so important? Here are some key factors that may help you understand why water is your essential life-force.

• 75% of Americans are chronically dehydrated.

• In 37% of Americans, the thirst mechanism is so weak that it is mistaken for hunger.

• Even MILD dehydration can slow down one's metabolism as much as 3%.

• One 8 ounce glass of water consumed before each meal will help decrease appetite and you will eat less.

- One glass of water may shut down midnight hunger for almost 100% of the dieters studied in a University of Washington study.

- If you don't drink enough water, your body may actually store water in response to your body's survival mechanism and you may not see the results you had expected on the scale.

- When your body breaks down fat reserve, water helps the kidneys remove the waste produced from the excess fat reserve and eliminate it from the body.

- Water assists in the excretion of waste from the bowel and kidneys and may help prevent constipation which is common with high protein diets.

- Lack of water is the number 1 cause of daytime fatigue.

- Water assists in digestion and the absorption of nutrients in food so while on a low calorie diet you will maintain the proper nourishment needed to your tissues and organs.

These tips should be convincing enough that drinking water is one of the key elements to achieving successful weight loss. If you have difficulty drinking water or find that it is just not satisfying, then try adding lemon or make iced tea instead. Herbal teas are a natural diuretic and highly recommended while on the HCG Diet Protocol. In summary, to maintain optimal health and to assist in managing your weight, drink more water. Consider keeping a bottle of water by your side at work, on your nightstand and in the car.

Why Do You Need a Food Journal?

Dieters who have made the commitment to do the hCG diet protocol must always remember that consistency is the key element. Keeping records in a journal daily will be the dieter's most important tool on the 800 Calorie Protocol.

Dieters should always be honest. If a dieter is not honest in their own personal journal, the only one they will be hurting and hiding the truth from is their own self.

Dieters should clearly define what their realistic goals are while on the 800 Calorie Protocol and record them at the beginning of their journal.

Dieters should make a list of excuses they tell themselves.

Dieters should write out a plan. Dieters will have a hard time sticking with the 800 Calorie Protocol if they do not have a plan. It is recommended that dieters plan for a week in advance. You are encouraged to think about everything going on within that week and plan accordingly. When dieters plan a week in advance, they are more likely to be successful. They should never deviate away from the plan once they have it. When they stray from the plan they should make note of that in their journal. Dieters should write about the people they were around and the situations they were in. They will be able to look back and access these details in the future to help them deal with similar circumstances.

The dieter's daily morning weigh in should always be recorded. This will give the dieter motivation and empowerment during different phases of the 800 Calorie Protocol.

Dieters should write down the details of every meal, snacks or beverages. This will be very helpful if the dieter needs to reference back and pinpoint certain items that may have caused increased losses or stalls. Food journaling also makes the dieter aware of their unconscious food habits. Once a dieter sees it written down, they can reflect on it and address it. Sometimes people tend to eat unconsciously. The simple act of writing it down brings the dieter a sharper focus of what they are consuming.

Dieters should write down those times they may stray from the 800 Calorie Protocol whether accidental or on purpose. They should write down how it happened, why it happened and how they felt afterwards. This will help to avoid any future mishaps.

It is important that the dieter feels good about their successes and acknowledges those successes as well. This will keep them on track physically as well as psychologically.

Dieters should always record how they are feeling in their journals. They may discover there are certain behaviors or emotions that contribute to poor eating habits or bad lifestyle decisions. Writing how they are feeling will help pinpoint triggers of when a dieter may make an unhealthy decision.

Questions & Answers

WHY 800 CALORIES AND NOT 500?

Answer: Experience suggests that your body must be in deprivation or starvation mode (less than 800 calories) in order for the HCG hormone to release abnormal fat reserves. This is why following a less than 800 calorie daily diet is just as effective as a 500 calorie restriction. Additionally, I have found that my patients have been able to tolerate an 800 calorie daily allowance more effectively and complete the 6 week course successfully. If you follow the sample guide and number of food choice servings, you should not go below 550 calories or above 800. I recommend about 725-750 calories per day. If you eat below 500 calories, your body may store the fat and you will not lose weight, rather you may gain!

WHY WAS DR. SIMEONS' ORIGINAL PROTOCOL MODIFIED?

Answer: There are some reputable medical organizations that say a 500-calorie daily diet–if not supervised–can be dangerous for the patient. Dr. Simeons created his protocol in the 1950s when we didn't have as much information about the human body and how it operates as we do now. Dr. Simeons closely monitored his patients daily in his office. That is next to impossible in today's modern weight management practices. Dr. Simeons' protocol would not allow breakfast. Breakfast is essential because it helps to increase the metabolic set point for the rest of the day. Dr. Simeons did not allow his patients to take their prescribed medications or the use of vitamins and minerals. Dieters should never stop their prescribed medication unless authorized by their physician. We also know that vitamins and minerals are the spark plugs of the human body. Supplying the tissues, organs, and cells with adequate nutrition will greatly enhance weight loss results. The additional 300 calories are derived mainly from protein which allows the dieter a more tolerable program to follow with a reduced frequency of headaches, weakness, and fatigue.

CAN I FOLLOW THE 800 CALORIE PROTOCOL IF I AM TAKING hCG DROPS?

Absolutely! HCG drops dieters are encouraged to follow the safer 800 calorie protocol that allows breakfast, the use of vitamins and minerals, and suggests continuing all prescribed medications. Remember to obtain approval from your physician before starting any restricted calorie diet.

WHY SHOULD I TAKE ESSENTIAL FATTY ACIDS WHILE ON THE HCG DIET?

Answer: There are only two EFAs: alpha-linolenic acid (omega-3) and linoleic acid (omega-6). EFAs are the "good fats" that the body cannot synthesize and can only be obtained through diet. Essential fatty acids help support the cardiovascular, reproductive, immune, and nervous systems. They are especially needed while on a restricted calorie intake.

CAN I CHEW GUM?

Answer: Yes, you may chew sugar free or an organic chewing gum. You may find this at most organic and whole food stores. Gum containing Xylitol is allowed but please remember that moderation is the key.

CAN I DRINK ALCOHOL WHILE ON PHASE 2?

Answer: No. You should not drink any alcohol as it contains many calories and carbohydrates. You may have 3-4 ounces of dry red organic wine in Phase 1.

CAN I ADD SALT TO MY FOOD IN PHASE 2?

Answer: You may use Sea Salt in Phase 2. However, please use it very sparingly. You may use lemon juice, apple cider raw unfiltered vinegar, ground pepper, parsley, oregano, and thyme for flavor on your proteins, vegetables and salad. See the approved condiments section in this book.

WHY DO I NEED TO EAT MY FAVORITE FOODS ON THE FIRST 2 LOADING DAYS IN PHASE 2?

Answer: You should eat your favorite fat and carbohydrate rich foods on the first 2 days of Phase 2 (Load day 1 and 2). This helps to build your fat stores before starting a restricted low calorie diet of 800 daily. It is not recommended to eat too much to where you feel sick and bloated. You may incorporate cooking oils, sugar and starches, all of which may be included in your 2 loading days. It takes about 3 days for the HCG to access abnormal fat reserves. In my experience, those who do not load will generally lose less weight. Please load up on all your favorite foods on these 2 days.

Recommended Loading Foods:

Nuts – walnuts, macadamia, cashews.

Fats/Oils - Mayo, avocados, coconut oil, butter, peanut butter

Dairy - Ice cream, heavy creams blended with fruit and drink it, half and half creamer, whole milk, whipping cream, whole eggs soaked in butter

Starches w/ FAT - Pasta with heavy alfredo sauce, bread and butter, bagels with cream cheese and butter, potato skins or baked potato with cheddar cheese, sour cream, bacon and loads of butter, shredded beef chimi's with flour tortilla, bean burritos.

All Deep Fried Foods - onion rings, chili cheese French fries with sour cream

Sweets - Turtle Cheesecake, peanut butter, éclairs, donuts, cupcakes, pastries, candy bars, pies, cakes.

Meat - Greasy bacon cheeseburgers, rib eye steak, sausage, pork spare ribs, rump roast, bacon.

DO I NEED TO EAT ALL ORGANIC FOODS?

Answer: It is recommended to eat all organic products, especially your proteins. Non-organic poultry, vegetables, fruit, and beef may contain preservatives, antibiotics, herbicides, pesticides, and flavor enhancers. If you do not have access to all organic foods, wash all produce thoroughly and do not drink tap water.

WHAT CAN I DO IF MY WEIGHT PLATEAUS?

Answer: It is very common for both men and women to have a 2-4 day weight plateau on any weight loss program. On the 4th day, you may eat only 6 green apples for the entire day and decrease your fluid intake by half. This is because your body may be retaining water. Another plateau breaker is fasting for the entire day by only drinking fluids and then eating a large steak 8-10 oz. for dinner. Both of these plateau breakers have had great results and the average weight loss is around 2 pounds overnight. You may also be constipated from being on a high protein diet. It is possible to hold 5 or more pounds of stool in your colon. We recommend taking an over the counter laxative to aid in digestion. (See Stall Breakers)

WOULD I LOSE THE SAME WEIGHT EATING A LOW CALORIE DIET WITHOUT THE HCG?

Answer: You can lose weight by simply eating fewer calories and fat. However, because the body stores fat during times of deprivation, you might lose muscle before fat in addition to a slower metabolism. Many people find that they will lose the weight but then gain it all back plus more! HCG alone will not help you lose the weight; rather a combination of the HCG medication, low impact daily exercise, proper nutrition, and a low calorie diet will help you to achieve your weight loss goals. Finally you can say goodbye to rollercoaster dieting once and for all.

WHAT HAPPENS IF I FORGET TO TAKE THE HCG?

Answer: The HCG remains in your body for about 3 days. It is best to take the HCG as soon as you wake up. However, if you forget and don't remember until several hours later, you may simply take the HCG at that time. If you skip an entire day, do not double your dose the next day.

IS THE HCG MADE FROM THE URINE OF PREGNANT WOMEN?

Answer: Yes, Human Chorionic Gonadotropin is a glycoprotein hormone that is extracted from the urine of pregnant women and is tested for potency and standardized by a biological assay procedure. It is the very same product given to women in high doses to induce fertilization.

WILL HCG INTERFERE WITH ANY MEDICATIONS I AM CURRENTLY TAKING?

Answer: No, HCG is not contraindicated with any medications. Please continue ALL medications prescribed to you by your medical doctor.

WHEN IS THE BEST TIME FOR A MENSTRUATING WOMAN TO START PHASE 2?

Answer: It is recommended to start the hCG medication at least 10 days before you are going to start your menstruation. You must stop the HCG medication as soon as your period begins. When you notice only a small amount of spotting (about 3 or 4 days later depending on your cycle), you may resume the medication. The increase in your hormone levels may cause you to bleed more heavily than normal or you may skip your period entirely. For dieters with a light menstrual flow, you may continue the hCG medication throughout the course of your menses.

WILL I SPOT EVEN THOUGH I AM POST MENOPAUSAL?

Answer: Some post-menopausal women have reported a small amount of spotting while taking HCG. This is the body's reaction to an increase of hormone production and is not considered a health concern.

WHY IS IT NECESSARY TO DO A PRE-DIET TOTAL BODY COLON CLEANSE IN PHASE 1 or 2?

Answer: Cleansing and detoxifying the colon is important to maintain general digestive health. Toxins can build up in your colon over a period of months and years. We are also exposed to a vast number of toxins in our food, the air, the water we drink, at the workplace and even in our homes. It is important to cleanse the colon in order to maintain digestive health.

IS IT TRUE THAT I CAN'T WEAR MAKEUP OR USE LOTION ON MY SKIN WHILE ON PHASE 2?

Answer: Dr. Simeons suggested that wearing makeup and oily skin products could possibly prevent weight loss. However, there is no data that we could find to support this concept. Tens of thousands of HCG dieters have used products that contained oil and did not report weight loss issues. Also, it is important to remember that 50 years ago there were higher concentrations of oils and animal fats in the products .However, if you desire to be oil-free, try Corn Huskers Oil Free Skin and Body Lotion.

WHAT IS A PHASE 2 'PLANNED INTERRUPTION'?

If an occasion arises that you need to take a break from the 800 Calorie Protocol, you may need to take a 'planned interruption'. Dr. Simeons suggests doing this until after your 20th day. Understand that you will most likely gain some weight but when you resume the protocol this weight will come off again. Be very careful and be sure to make wise choices during this interruption. You do not want to gain unnecessary weight or re-gain the pounds you've worked so hard to lose.

You can plan an interruption for up to a maximum of 2 weeks. You must stop the hcg 3 days before and stay on the 800 Calorie Protocol. Then you may increase your calories by eating P3 foods only. Do not eat any sugar or starches during your interruption and maintain no more than 1500 calories daily. When your interruption has ended, you may resume the hcg and finish out your round.

Chapter 6

Phase 3 Stabilization - 3 Weeks

Most Important Phase! Please follow carefully

After you have completed 72 hours without hCG in Phase 2, you will now begin Phase 3. You must increase your calories in this phase. In Phase 3, your body no longer has the hCG working to protect your lean muscle. During Phase 3, it is very important to maintain lean muscle tissue to prevent a slowed metabolism.

This plan was developed to add in allowable fats and jump right up to 1500 calories on P3, day one. This can be safely carried out, without the possibility of gaining weight, due to the omission of nuts, breads, beans, legumes, and limiting dairy. However, most dieters prefer to slowly add back in their calories and that is fine. For dieters who want to stabilize at their new weight, during the next 3 weeks you must keep your weight within +/- 2 pounds of where you were when you stopped taking HCG. This will allow your hypothalamus to reset and establish your new weight as your normal weight. If you gain more than 2lbs, you may do a correction day (depending on the cause of gain). If you lose more than 2lbs, increase your food intake by 100-200 calories.

To gradually increase your calories when following the 500 or 800 calorie protocols, you may refer to the guide below:

WEEK 1: 900-1100 calories per day
WEEK 2: 1100-1300 calories per day
WEEK 3: 1300-1500 calories per day

WEEK 1:
900-1100 calories per day.

Work up to your estimated caloric need by beginning at 900 calories for this 7 day period and gradually increase your calories to reach 1100 by the end of week 1.

WEEK 2:
1100-1300 calories per day.

Work up to your estimated caloric need by beginning at 1100 calories for this 7 day period and gradually increase your calories to reach 1300 by the end of week 2.

By week 2, if you haven't already, you can start adding healthy oil fats such as avocados, cooking oils, whole eggs, and low moisture, skim mozzarella cheese. Full fats are allowed such as full fat, no sugar, salad dressing and mayonnaise. (Please make sure to observe the sugar and caloric content.) Some dieters may choose to add these back in the first week, just make sure you watch the scale and don't overdo it. We recommend to obtain optimal stabilization, especially if this is your last round, to hold off on adding in nuts, grain breads (sprouted or un-sprouted - aka, Ezekiel bread), beans, legumes, and limit dairy in the 21 days of stabilization. All too often people over-indulge on these items which can stress out the adrenals and engage a whole chain reaction leading to weight gain.

* If you MUST have nuts (which is NOT recommended) you must limit it to 1 serving per day (about 10-15 pieces)

WEEK 3:

1300-1500 calories per day.

Work up to your estimated caloric need by beginning at 1300 calories for this 7 day period and gradually increase your calories to reach 1500 by the end of week 3.

Please keep in mind that everyone's body is unique. Some foods that may be agreeable to others may not be agreeable to you. You are encouraged to keep track of your food intake with the tracker provided on a daily basis. This way, if you have any issues during Phase 3, you can go back and pinpoint what food item(s) may have caused this.

- Increase your protein to about 6 oz. per serving.

- Continue to drink plenty of water daily.

- Increase your daily caloric intake to about 1500-2300 calories. Learn how to estimate your caloric daily intake by using our simple calculation method. (see next page)

- You may have any fruit or vegetable you wish except corn, yams, and bananas (in moderation) as they are high in sugar and carbohydrates.

- You may eat any kind of meat, fish, shellfish, or poultry desired.

- You may use extra virgin olive oil, organic coconut oil, or MCT oil in moderation.

- You may eat cheese but only low moisture skim mozzarella and very sparingly in this 21 day period.

- Continue to avoid butter and margarine.

- Seasonings may be used that are low in sodium.

- Limit dairy products if possible.

- Avoid nuts, breads, beans, and legumes.

- Continue to avoid sweets.

During this period, the "starchy" carbohydrates, such as sugar, rice, bread, potatoes, pasta, pastries, etc., should be avoided. Other foods to avoid are nuts, legumes, cereal, granola bars, protein bars (unless low in sugar and carbohydrates), and oatmeal. I recommend healthy carbohydrates from fruits and vegetables, and good fats obtained from specific oils. If you shock your body quickly and load up on complex carbohydrates, the potential for weight gain is possible. This must be carefully observed during the first 3 weeks (21 days) after the treatment has ended, otherwise, you may gain a few pounds back and your metabolism may not reset properly.

After the initial 3-week period, you can start adding back in complex carbohydrates in moderation to your diet, one at a time, during the following 3 weeks. The reason for adding only 1 new food item at a time (1 per day) is so that you can determine the following day if that food agrees or doesn't agree with your body system, based on the feedback from your scale. A sudden increase in weight may mean you have eaten something that is causing inflammation or water retention in your body and you might want to consider avoiding that food, or having a smaller serving of it, in the future.

Try to eat six times per day. It is very important to eat breakfast, lunch, and dinner, and have three snacks throughout the day. This will promote an increase in metabolism. You may exercise more aggressively now, as your body is taking in a higher amount of calories.

Resistance training is acceptable in this phase as tolerated and you may increase the length of your cardio workouts as tolerated. If you need to lose more weight, you must remain on Phase 3 for an additional 3 weeks for a total of 6 weeks until you start your second round of the HCG. The new protocol requires the prescribing physician to inform the patient that a 6 week break is required before starting another round.

Phase 3 Correction Days

Phase 3 was designed to assure your new stabilized weight by removing the foods that many over-indulge upon. Correction days are seldom needed when following this plan. A correction day is not to be utilized to justify cheating or planning a cheat day, rather it is to bring down an unknown gain or an accidental mishap. I do understand that mishaps may occur so I have listed my approved correction day methods if you have gained more than 2 pounds from your last dose weight (LDW).

* For women, do not attempt to utilize a correction day if your menstrual cycle has caused your weight to go above 2 pounds from your LDW. This is natural water retention and will eventually flush out when your menstrual cycle has ended.

Non-Fat Fage Yogurt Correction Day

Non-fat 0% Plain Greek yogurt contains probiotics that help to reduce intestinal inflammation, water retention, and bloating.

Brands allowed: Plain Fage, All Natural Brown Cow Plain, and Dannon Oikos Plain

(Plain Greek Yogurt only with NO added fruit)

Directions: #2- 16 oz. tubs or #1- 32 oz. tub of approved 0% NON FAT PLAIN Greek Yogurt, divide into **8 oz.** servings and add 2 oz. of fresh berries per serving (fresh strawberries or raspberries are preferred.) Eat 4 servings throughout the day. Your total caloric daily value is estimated at about 800-850 calories. Continue drinking your regular daily fluids.

Dr. Simeons "Steak Day"

Directions: Drink plenty of fluids all day long and do not eat anything until dinner. When you can, eat a large steak cooked in oil or butter with an apple or a raw tomato. The next day, you should see your weight drop.

* Fasting all day is not so healthy for you, so the "steak day" should only be utilized for those that are unable to tolerate plain Greek yogurt.

* If you have issues with low blood sugar, you are permitted an apple for lunch, as per Dr. Simeons.

Sodium Overload

If you have mistakenly overindulged in a high sodium food product that has caused a gain above your 2 pound limit, you may consider this natural remedy to remove excess sodium and toxins.

Detox Bath

1 cup Epsom salt
1 cup Sea salt (non-iodized)
2 cups Baking soda

Directions: Run a bath as hot as you can stand and soak for 20 minutes. You may wash your body with plain glycerin soap. Be sure to drink plenty of cold water while you are submerged in the tub, as an increase in sweating is expected. If you do not drink plenty of fluids, you may experience a slight headache.

Hot Lemon Water Detox

2 lemons
Stevia

Directions: Drink an 8 oz. cup of hot water with the juice of half a lemon 4 times throughout the day. Add Stevia to sweeten if desired. Make sure your last cup of the day is right at bedtime.

Calculating your Phase 3 Caloric Intake

The best way to maintain your weight loss is first to understand that everyone's body size, shape, and weight differs. An easy equation to calculate your estimated total caloric intake for the day will be your baseline to achieve maximum weight management.

Women must multiply their weight by 12 and men by 13.

For example:

Women

140 (pounds) X **12** = 1680 calories per day to maintain weight loss.

Men

180 (pounds) X **13** = 2340 calories per day to maintain weight loss.

Try to exercise at least 3 times per week, take your daily vitamins and supplements, and drink plenty of water.

Phase 3 Sample Menu (Female)

Sample Goal Menu for *Female* 130 Lbs.
(Refer to high protein diet guide and calorie chart)

	Calories	Protein	Carbs.	Fat	Sodium
Breakfast					
(1 protein and 1 fruit choice)					
1 scoop *Protein Powder* *(optional)*	120.0	23.0	3.0	3.0	150.00
3 egg whites	51.0	10.5	0.6	0.3	164.25
4 tsp. olive oil	159.0	-	-	18	-
1 small banana	89.0	0.9	18.5	-	0.8
Totals:	**419.0**	**34.4**	**22.1**	**21.3**	**315.05**
Morning Snack *(1 protein)*					
4 oz. low-fat cottage cheese	80.0	15.0	4.0	2.0	460.0
Totals:	**80.0**	**15.0**	**4.0**	**2.0**	**460.0**
Lunch					
(1 protein, 1 vegetable and 1 fruit choice)					
3 oz. chicken breast, *cooked*	148.0	21.0	-	1.0	71.25
4 tsp. olive oil	159.0	-	-	18.0	-
6 oz. broccoli	60.0	5.0	9.0	-	29.0
1 small orange	45.0	0.9	11.3	0.1	-
Totals:	**412.0**	**26.9**	**20.3**	**19.1**	**100.25**

Afternoon Snack *(fruit choice)*					
1 small grapefruit or ½ large grapefruit	32.0	0.6	8.1	0.1	-
Totals:	**32.0**	**0.6**	**8.1**	**0.1**	-
Dinner *(1 protein, 1 vegetable, and salad)*					
4 oz. swordfish	175.0	27.5	-	5.0	130.0
4 tsp. olive oil	159.0	-	-	18.0	-
6 oz. asparagus	48.0	6.0	7.0	1.0	3.0
Totals:	**382.0**	**33.5**	**7.0**	**24.0**	**133.0**
Salad					
3 oz. lettuce	11.0	0.5	2.4	-	7.5
2 oz. tomato	12.0	0.6	2.5	-	1.6
2 oz. cucumber	8.0	0.3	2	-	3.3
2 oz. celery	9.0	-	2.6	-	26
1 tsp. apple cider vinegar	4.0	-	2.3	-	-
Totals:	**44.0**	**1.4**	**11.8**	-	**38.4**
Evening Snack *(Optional)*					
2 oz. mozzarella cheese (part-skim)	170.0	14.6	2.2	11.2	147.0
TOTALS:	**170.0**	**14.6**	**2.2**	**11.2**	**147.0**
Grand Totals:	**1,539**	**106.4**	**76.04**	**77.7**	**1,193.7**

Phase 3 Sample Menu (Male)

Sample Goal Menu for *Male* 180 Lbs.
(Refer to high protein diet guide and calorie chart)

	Calories	Protein	Carbs	Fat	Sodium
Breakfast *(1 protein and 1 fruit choice)*					
1 scoop *Protein Powder* *(optional)*	120.0	23.0	3.0	3.0	150.0
3 oz. turkey sausage	169.0	12.0	1.0	12.0	746.0
4 tsp. olive oil	159.0	-	-	18.0	-
1 cup grapes	110.0	1.2	29.0	0.3	3.2
TOTALS:	**558.0**	**36.2**	**33.0**	**31.3**	**899.0**

	Calories	Protein	Carbs	Fat	Sodium
Morning Snack *(1 protein choice)*					
6 oz. white tuna *(canned in water)*	210.0	45.0	-	1.0	190.0
Totals:	**210.0**	**45.0**	**-**	**1.0**	**190.0**

	Calories	Protein	Carbs	Fat	Sodium
Lunch *(1protein, 1 vegetable, and 1 fruit choice)*					
6 oz. lean meat *(chuck steak)*	324.0	42.0	-	32.0	130.0
4 tsp. olive oil	159.0	-	-	18.0	-
6 oz. mushrooms	48.0	2.0	8.0	-	25.0
1 small pear	81.0	0.5	21.5	0.2	1.5
TOTALS:	**612.0**	**44.5**	**29.5**	**40.2**	**156.5**

Afternoon Snack *(fruit choice)*					
1 cup blueberries	83.0	1.1	21.0	0.5	1.5
TOTALS:	83.0	1.1	21.0	0.5	1.5
Dinner *(1 protein, 1 vegetable, and salad)*					
6 oz. chicken *no skin*	282.0	42.0	-	4.0	114.0
6 oz. carrots	71.0	2.0	16.0	-	80.0
1 tsp. olive oil	40.0	-	4.6	4.5	-
TOTALS:	393.0	44.0	20.6	8.5	194.0
Salad					
3 oz. lettuce	11.0	0.5	2.4	-	7.5
2 oz. tomato	12.0	0.6	2.5	-	1.6
2 oz. cucumber	8.0	0.3	2.0	-	3.3
2 oz. celery	9.0	-	2.6	-	26.0
1 tsp. olive oil	40.	-	4.6	4.5	-
1 tsp. balsamic vinegar	7.0	-	3	-	-
TOTALS:	87.0	1.4	17.1	4.5	38.4
Evening Snack *(optional)*					-
2 oz. Mozzarella part-skim cheese	170.0	14.6	2.2	11.2	147.0
TOTALS:	170.0	14.6	2.2	11.2	147.0
GRAND TOTALS:	2,113	188.8	123.4	97.2	1,626.4

Phase 3 Calorie Counting

Beverages

Water – flavored

Crystal Light	5 cal
Herbal Tea – unsweetened	0 cal
Lifewater	0 cal
Zevia - diet cola	0 cal

Lean Meat Serving size 1 oz.

Top Sirloin Steak	62 cal /oz.
Extra Lean Hamburger	48 cal
London Broil	52 cal
Chuck Steak	54 cal
Veal	61 cal
Lean Bison	49 cal
Lamb	52 cal

Shellfish

Clams	41 cal
Lobster	28 cal
Mussels	48 cal

Oysters	19 cal
Scallops	23 cal
Shrimp	22 cal
Crab	31 cal

Fish

Bass	41 cal
Bluefish	45 cal
Cod	29 cal
Grouper	33 cal
Halibut	31 cal
Herring	39 cal
Mackerel	74 cal
Orange Roughy	29 cal
Red Snapper	36 cal
Salmon	51 cal
Shark	50 cal
Tilapia	42 cal
Trout	53 cal
Tuna	52 cal
Mahi-Mahi	37 cal

Dairy & Eggs

Skim Milk (1 cup)	85 cal
1% Low Fat Milk (1 cup)	110 cal
2% Low Fat Milk (1 cup)	122 cal
Whole Milk (1 cup)	150 cal
Almond Milk (1 cup) *unsweetened	40 cal
Coconut Milk (1 cup) *unsweetened	50 cal
Whole Egg (1 large)	80 cal
Mozzarella Part Skim (1 oz)	72 cal
Cottage Cheese (4 oz) 100 cal *less than 140mg of sodium	
Plain Greek Yogurt (1 cup) *0 % non-fat	80 cal
Plain Greek Yogurt (1cup) *2%	170 cal

Fruits

Apple (1 small)	55 cal
Apricot (4 small)	64 cal
Banana (1 small)	89 cal
Blackberries (1 cup)	74 cal
Blueberries (1 cup)	81 cal
Boysenberries (1 cup)	66 cal
Cantaloupe (1 cup)	54 cal

Cranberries (1 cup)	43 cal
Grapes (1 cup)	62 cal
Guava (1 cup)	112 cal
Honeydew Melon (1 cup)	61 cal
Kiwi (2 small)	92 cal
Mango (1/2 small)	67 cal
Peach (1small)	50 cal
Raspberries (1 cup)	60 cal
Strawberries (1 cup)	43 cal
Watermelon (1 cup)	70 cal

Cooking Oils

1 Tbsp *can vary by brand

Coconut Oil	120 cal
Olive Oil Extra Virgin	120 cal
MCT Oil	115 cal
Canola Oil	120 cal

Lean Poultry per oz.

Chicken Breast (white meat)	47 cal
Turkey Breast (white meat)	48 cal.

Vegetables *calories per 6 oz.*

Brussels Sprouts	48 cal
Cabbage	138 cal
Artichoke	126 cal
Asparagus	59 cal
Broccoli	60 cal
Cauliflower	37 cal
Celery	42 cal
Collards	49 cal
Cucumber	30 cal
Eggplant	90 cal
Endive	36 cal
Green Onions	36 cal
Kale	48 cal
Lettuce (green)	30 cal
Mushrooms	42 cal
Peppers (all varieties)	50 cal
Spinach	41 cal
Tomato	30 cal
Turnips	40 cal
Watercress	22 cal

Phase 3 HCG Recipes

Phase 3- Condiments

Avocado Dip - Great for dipping Veggies
5 avocados
2 cups of cottage cheese
2 cups of salsa *(refer to salsa recipe)*
½ juice of lemon
1 tsp. garlic powder
½ tsp. cumin
¼ cup cilantro
Sea salt and black pepper optional for taste

Cut avocadoes into chunks and place into a large bowl. Add cottage cheese. Add salsa, draining juice from salsa first. Squeeze juice from lemon into mixture. Add garlic powder and cumin. Hand mix lightly to keep mixture chunky. Add in cilantro, sea salt and black pepper for taste.

Creamy Dressing - Great on salads or use as a flavor enhancer on proteins
1 tsp. black ground pepper
½ tsp. of celery seed
½ tsp. dried dill
2 tsp. onion powder
2 cups of mayonnaise

Mix all ingredients together in a medium sized mixing bowl. Refrigerate. Let dressing sit for at least 6 hours for flavoring.

Cocktail Sauce
1/4 cup of ketchup *(refer to ketchup recipe)*
1 tsp. horseradish
1 T lemon juice
Sea salt and black pepper optional for taste

Mix ingredients together. Add more horseradish, sea salt and black pepper as needed for desired taste.

HCG Ketchup
1 can of organic no sugar added tomato sauce
2 T onion powder
½ tsp. sea salt
½ tsp. vinegar
1 tsp. paprika
1/8 tsp. cinnamon
2 packets of Stevia

Mix all ingredients thoroughly in a medium sized mixing bowl. Store in a plastic squeeze bottle and refrigerate.

Meat or No Meat Tomato Sauce
10 medium to large tomatoes
1 large onion
4 cloves of garlic
2 T oregano
¼ cup extra virgin olive oil

Slice onion and place in a food processor or blender until minced. Add olive oil to a large skillet and heat on medium heat. When oil is hot, add minced onion and cook until onions are clear. Add garlic and reduce heat. Chop tomatoes into a blender or food processor. Pulse tomatoes for 30 seconds. Add tomatoes and oregano and simmer 30-45 minutes until sauce thickens.

Meat Tomato Sauce

1 lb. of meat of your choice

Cook meat thoroughly and add to recipe after adding tomatoes and oregano.

Barbecue Sauce

1 ½ cups of no meat tomato sauce *(refer to recipe)*
2 large onions, minced
3 T lemon juice
1 tsp. sea salt
1 tsp. paprika
1tsp chili powder
¼ tsp. black ground pepper
¼ tsp. cinnamon
1/8 tsp. cloves

Combine all ingredients in a large cooking pot. Cover and heat on low for 35-45minutes, occasionally stirring. Refrigerate when done.

Spicy Salsa

2 tomatoes, diced
1 large red onion
3 T minced garlic
½ of a fresh jalapeno
1 cup of cilantro
Sea salt and black pepper optional for taste

Add all ingredients in a blender and pulse for 30 seconds. Add sea salt and black pepper for desired taste.

Taco Seasoning

4 T chili powder
1 T garlic powder
1 T onion powder
1 T dried oregano
1 T basil
2 T paprika
5 T ground cumin
1 T sea salt
1 T black pepper
½ T crushed red pepper flakes

Mix all ingredients thoroughly and store in an air tight container. Use 1-2 tablespoons per pound of desired meat.

Phase 3 - Soups & Salads

Bacon and Broccoli Salad
1 bag of thawed and drained frozen broccoli
½ cup shredded low moisture mozzarella cheese
½ pound of cooked and crumbled bacon
1 cup ranch dressing
½ cup chopped scallions
¼ tsp. ground black pepper
¼ tsp. sea salt

Mix all ingredients in a large mixing bowl. Chill in refrigerator at least 3 hours before serving.

Chicken BLT Salad
4 boneless chicken breasts grilled and cut in cubes
8 cups lettuce, chopped
2 cups cherry tomatoes
1 cup shredded low moisture mozzarella cheese
½ lb. of cooked and crumbled bacon
2 boiled eggs, chopped
1 cup ranch dressing
½ tsp. ground black pepper
¼ tsp. parsley

Separate lettuce on 4 serving plates. Add all ingredients in a large mixing bowl and mix thoroughly. Serve equal portions on bed of lettuce.

Chicken Salad
4 grilled boneless chicken breasts cut in cubes
4 celery stalks, chopped
1 cup of mayonnaise
½ tsp. sea salt
½ tsp. ground black pepper
2 T chives, chopped
½ cup dill pickles, chopped

Mix all ingredients thoroughly in a large mixing bowl. Refrigerate for 2 hours.

Marinated Tomatoes
1 lb. tomatoes cut in quarters
½ cup scallions, chopped
3 T parsley
¼ cup red wine vinegar
½ cup olive oil
1 T seasoning salt
1 T garlic salt
1 package of Stevia

Set tomatoes to the side. Mix all ingredients together. Toss in tomatoes and let sit at room temperature for 3 hours. Drain excess marinate and serve.

Tuna Salad
2 Tuna, drained
2 cups cherry tomatoes cut in halves
¼ cup scallions, chopped
½ cup mayonnaise
¼ tsp. dill weed
½ tsp. ground black pepper
¼ tsp. sea salt
2 T parsley

Mix all ingredients in a large mixing bowl. Chill 2 hours in refrigerator before serving.

Asian Beef Soup
1 lb. organic grass fed beef
1 lb. head bok choy
1 large onion, chopped
½ cup scallions, chopped
1 clove of minced garlic
4 cups of chicken broth (if canned read label for starch)
2 T reduced sodium soy sauce
Ground black pepper

Chop the bok choy separating stalks and leaves. Lightly coat organic olive oil in a 4-6 quart soup pot. Over low heat, brown onions, mushrooms, scallions, garlic and beef. Drain any excess grease. Add bok choy stalks and cook until almost tender. Add soy sauce and broth and bring to a boil. Stir in the bok choy leaves and cook until heated through. Season with black, ground pepper for desired taste.

Chicken Vegetable Soup

2 grilled and cubed chicken breasts
½ cup celery, chopped
2 small yellow squash, chopped
5 large mushrooms, sliced
2 cans of chicken broth (*if canned read label for starch and sodium*)
1 tsp. chicken bouillon cube, crushed
½ cup bottled or filtered water
2 T parsley, chopped
¼ tsp. black ground pepper
¼ tsp. sea salt
2 T heavy cream

Lightly coat organic olive oil in a 4-6 quart soup pot over low heat. Add all vegetables and cook approximately 5 minutes. Add chicken, broth, bouillon, bottled or filtered water, parsley, pepper, sea salt, and simmer uncovered for 10- 15 minutes. Add heavy cream. Then serve.

Goulash Soup
2 lbs. sirloin beef, cubed
1 large onion, chopped
3 minced cloves of garlic
2 T paprika
14 ½ oz. no sugar added tomatoes, diced
4 beef bouillon cubes *(low in sodium)*
1tsp of Stevia
½ tsp. marjoram
½ tsp. ground black pepper
1 zucchini, diced
1 green pepper, chopped
1 can of beef broth *(check label for starch and sodium)*
6 cups of bottled or filtered water
In a 4-6 quart soup pot

Lightly coat organic olive oil in a 4-6 quart soup pot over low heat. Brown beef, onion and garlic. Add paprika and stir to coat beef. Add remaining ingredients EXCEPT the zucchini and green pepper. Bring to a boil. Cover and simmer for 1 hour until beef is tender. Add zucchini and green pepper and simmer another 20 minutes.

Mushroom and Broccoli Soup
16 oz. of cooked broccoli
½ cup of heavy cream
½ cup bottled or filtered water
½ lb. mushrooms, sliced
14 oz. can beef broth *(check label for starch)*
½ tsp. ground black pepper
1 tsp. sea salt
1 minced garlic clove
1T minced onion

Lightly coat organic olive oil in a 4-6 quart pot. Preheat over low heat. Cook mushrooms, onion, garlic and seasonings until lightly brown. Add beef broth, bottled or filtered water and broccoli and bring to a boil. Cover and cook approximately 8 minutes or until the broccoli is tender. Puree with a hand held blender until smooth and then add in heavy cream and stir.

Tomato Bisque

2 cans of organic tomatoes
1 8oz. package of low moisture, skim Mozzarella cheese
2 tsp. basil
2 tbsp. heavy cream
1 package of Stevia
1/8 tsp. hot pepper flakes
¼ tsp. ground black pepper
¼ tsp. sea salt

Lightly coat organic olive oil in a 4-6 quart pot. Preheat over low heat. Cook tomatoes and spices for 5 minutes. Add Mozzarella cheese. Use hand mixer and blend. Add heavy cream and stir.

Phase 3 – Appetizers & Snacks

Deviled Eggs
8 hard-boiled eggs
½ cup of mayonnaise
2 T minced onion
2 T minced celery
1 tsp. mustard
1/8 tsp. sea salt
1/8 ground black pepper
Pinch of celery salt
Paprika

Cut eggs in half and remove yolks from whites and place in a mixing bowl. Combine all ingredients EXCEPT paprika. Mix thoroughly until smooth. Fill the egg whites with yolk mixture and then sprinkle with paprika. Refrigerate.

Extra Protein Deviled Eggs
Add a 6oz. can of drained tuna to recipe above

Mushrooms with Crab Stuffing
1 cup shredded Alaskan king crab or snow crab
1 tsp. lemon juice
¼ tsp. basil
¼ tsp. garlic powder
½ cup minced scallions
1/8 tsp. lemon pepper
½ cup grated Mozzarella cheese
24 large mushrooms

Pre-heat oven to 450 degrees. Wash mushrooms and remove stems. Set mushroom caps aside. Finely chop 12 of the mushroom stems. In a large mixing bowl combine the 12 finely chopped mushroom stems, crab, lemon juice, basil, garlic powder, scallions, and lemon pepper. DO NOT ADD CHEESE at this point. Mix thoroughly. Coat a large baking dish with organic olive oil. Fill mushroom caps with mixture and place in baking dish. Top with grated Mozzarella cheese. Bake for 20 minutes.

Mozzarella Crusted Squash

2 medium yellow squash, sliced
1 egg
¼ cup grated Mozzarella cheese

Coat a medium skillet with organic olive oil. Preheat on low heat. Wisk one egg in a bowl. Place grated Mozzarella cheese on flat plate. Dip squash slices into egg and then coat with Mozzarella cheese. Fry in skillet until both sides are golden brown.

Pork Stuffed Mushrooms

24 large mushrooms
1 lb. of pork sausage
8 oz. shredded low moisture mozzarella cheese
Sea salt and pepper to desired taste

Preheat oven to 350 degrees. Wash mushrooms and remove stems. Place mushroom caps aside. Preheat large skillet over medium heat. Chop stems finely and place in skillet with pork sausage. Cook until sausage is thoroughly cooked. Drain excess fat. Coat large baking dish with organic olive oil. Combine remaining ingredients and mix well. Fill mushroom caps with mixture and place in baking dish. Bake for 25 minutes.

Meat Lovers Pizza
2 packages of mushrooms, sliced
2 green peppers, chopped
1 onion, chopped
1 ½ cups meatless tomato sauce (refer to recipe)
½ lb. cooked Italian sausage
½ lb. cooked chicken breast cut and cubed in small pieces
15 slices of pepperoni
½ cup of cooked bacon crumbled
1 cup shredded low moisture mozzarella cheese

Preheat oven to 400 degrees. Spray bottom of baking pan with organic olive oil. Arrange mushroom slices to cover bottom of the pan. Pour tomato sauce over the mushrooms. Add meats and vegetables in any order you prefer. Top with mozzarella cheese. Bake for 20 minutes.

Spinach Casserole
2 packages frozen spinach, thawed and chopped
2 cups cottage cheese
½ cup egg whites
½ cup grated mozzarella cheese
¼ tsp. ground black pepper
Paprika

Pre-heat oven to 375 degrees. Cook spinach until heated through. Drain thoroughly, squeezing out excess water. In a mixing bowl add cottage cheese, egg whites, ground black pepper and cheese. Mix thoroughly. Mix in spinach. Spray a 9 inch pie pan with organic olive oil cooking spray. Pour mixture into pie pan and sprinkle paprika and some additional mozzarella cheese. Bake for approximately 30 minutes or until firm and lightly browned at the edges.

Phase 3 - Breakfast

Banana Pancakes
1 banana
2 eggs
¾ tsp. vanilla extract
¼ tsp. cinnamon

Spray skillet with organic olive oil. Preheat skillet on low heat. Mix ingredients in a blender. Pulse 5-6 times. Pour batter in skillet. Cook slowly. Great with Berry Syrup *(see recipe below)*.

Berry Syrup
1 cup of fresh or frozen mixed berries. (strawberries, raspberries, blackberries, etc.)

Place berries in a microwave safe bowl. Microwave 1 to 1 ½ minutes on high. Mash with a fork and serve.

Bacon Cheese Quiche
6 eggs
2 tbsp. heavy cream
½ tsp. salt
¼ tsp. ground black pepper
¼ cup scallions, chopped
6 bacon slices, cooked
½ cup of shredded low moisture mozzarella

Preheat oven to 350 degrees. Lightly coat a large pie dish with organic olive oil. Combine eggs, cream and seasonings into mixing bowl and beat with a hand mixer. Pour mixture into pie plate. Place remaining ingredients on top. Bake 30-35 minutes.

Breakfast Stir-Fry
3 bacon slices, chopped
¼ cup onion, chopped
¼ cup green pepper, chopped
¼ cup red pepper, chopped
½ cup squash, chopped
2 eggs

Place bacon in a medium skillet. Cook bacon until it starts to brown and renders fat. Add onion, green pepper, red pepper and squash. Cook and stir over low heat until vegetables are tender and caramelized and bacon is cooked. Pour mixture onto serving plate. In same skillet fry 2 eggs and serve them over mixture.

Avocado Scrambler
2 eggs
½ red pepper, chopped
½ avocado, coarsely chopped
1 t grated mozzarella cheese
Sea salt
Ground black pepper

Spray small skillet with organic olive oil. Preheat on medium heat. Add eggs to skillet and break yolks. Add a dash of sea salt and ground black pepper. Stir to scramble and continue stirring until eggs start to firm up. Add peppers and avocado and cook until egg firmness is desired. Sprinkle mozzarella cheese.

Spinach Omelet

2 eggs
1 cup baby spinach, chopped
2 T grated mozzarella cheese
¼ tsp. onion powder
¼ tsp. basil
1/8 tsp. ground nutmeg
Sea salt and ground black pepper to taste

Lightly coat skillet with organic olive oil. In mixing bowl beat eggs and stir in baby spinach and mozzarella cheese. Season with basil, onion powder, nutmeg, sea salt and ground black pepper. Pour mixture into skillet and cook approximately 3 minutes until partially firm. Flip with spatula and continue cooking approximately 3 minutes or to desired texture.

Phase 3 - Chicken

Balsamic Grilled Chicken
8 (4 oz.) boneless skinless chicken breast
1 cup bottled or filtered water
½ cup olive oil
2 T balsamic vinegar
4 tsp. dried onion flakes
1 tsp. oregano
1 tsp. basil
1 tsp. parsley
3 tsp. ground mustard
2 tsp. thyme
2 tsp. sea salt
2 tsp. ground black pepper

Mix olive oil, balsamic vinegar, oregano, basil, parsley, thyme, salt, pepper, bottled or filtered water and onion flakes in 1 gallon re-sealable plastic bag along with chicken breast. Allow chicken to marinate for at least a half hour. Preheat grill on medium heat. Place chicken on grill and sear both sides. Grill until fully cooked.

BBQ Chicken
1 lb. boneless skinless chicken breasts
1 cup no sugar added barbecue sauce *(refer to recipe)*

In a zip-lock bag, combine chicken with barbecue sauce. Coat chicken evenly and marinate in the refrigerator for 2 hours. Heat grill to medium heat. Grill chicken until fully cooked.

Chicken Burgers

1 lb. of ground chicken
1 egg
¼ cup mushrooms, cooked and finely chopped
½ cup onion, finely diced
1 cup spinach leaves, finely shredded
½ tsp. sea salt
½ tsp. ground black pepper

Mix all ingredients into a large mixing bowl and hand mix. Shape mixture into 4 patties. Preheat grill on medium heat. Cook patties 5 minutes on each side or until fully cooked.

Chicken Fajitas

1 lb. boneless skinless chicken breasts cut into strips
4 tsp. sea salt
2 tsp. ground black pepper
2 tsp. cumin
2 tsp. chili powder
2 tsp. onion powder
2 tsp. garlic powder
1 cup of bottled or filtered water
2 green pepper, cut into strips
2 medium onion, thinly sliced
5 T lime juice
Salsa *(refer to recipe)*
Any allowed favorite toppings, lettuce, onions, tomatoes, black olives, etc.

In a zip-lock plastic bag combine the chili powder, salt, cumin, onion powder, ground black pepper, garlic powder, and bottled or filtered water. Add chicken, bell pepper and onion. Seal and knead gently to coat. Refrigerate for 15 minutes. Heat a large nonstick skillet on medium heat. Empty contents of bag into the skillet and cook. Stir occasionally until vegetables are crisp and tender and chicken is cooked through. Remove from heat. Serve.

Chicken Mozzarella

3 boneless skinless chicken breasts
1 cup onion, chopped
4 minced garlic cloves
3 cans of organic no sugar added diced tomatoes
1 T oregano
1 T basil
2 packages of Stevia
1 ½ cups shredded low moisture mozzarella cheese

Coat a large skillet with organic olive oil. Preheat over medium heat. Add chicken breast, onions, and garlic to hot skillet, brown on both sides. When both sides are browned, add tomatoes, Stevia, basil and oregano to the skillet. Move the chicken around in the tomato sauce to coat all sides. Cook on medium heat uncovered for thirty minutes. This will thicken the sauce. Spread the low moisture mozzarella on top of the entire skillet. Cover and cook until cheese is melted.

Chicken and Spinach

4 boneless skinless chicken breasts, pounded flat
1 tsp. sea salt
1 tsp. desired seasoning
½ pound mushrooms, quartered
2 minced garlic cloves
1 bag of baby spinach

Season chicken breasts with sea salt and desired seasoning on both sides. Grill chicken and set aside. Coat a large skillet with organic olive oil and preheat on medium heat. Sauté mushrooms and garlic until tender. Add spinach to skillet and cook until just wilted. Stir occasionally when cooking spinach to stir up mushrooms from the bottom of skillet. Serve spinach mixture over grilled chicken.

Crock Pot Chicken Tacos
1 lb. boneless skinless chicken breasts
2 cups of salsa *(refer to recipe)*
4 T taco seasoning *(refer to recipe)*
1 lime
4 T cilantro, chopped
Any allowed favorite toppings, lettuce, onions, peppers, black olives, etc.

Spray crock pot with organic olive oil. Add salsa, taco seasoning, cilantro and squeeze out the juice from lime. Stir mixture. Add chicken. Cook on low for 8-10 hours. Remove chicken and shred. Place on serving dish and add any of your allowed favorite toppings.

Chili Chicken
4 boneless skinless chicken breasts
2 T extra virgin olive oil
2 T cilantro
1 T chili powder
1 T cumin
2 tsp. sea salt
2 minced garlic cloves
1/8 tsp. cayenne pepper
¼ cup green pepper, chopped
3 T red onion, diced
¼ cup tomatoes, diced
½ cup low moisture mozzarella cheese

Preheat oven to 400 degrees. In a mixing bowl, add extra virgin olive oil, cilantro, chili powder, cumin, sea salt, minced garlic, and cayenne pepper. Add the chicken and rub mixture on breasts until coated evenly. Coat a baking dish with organic olive oil. Place chicken in baking dish. Arrange green peppers, onions, and tomatoes over the chicken. Bake for 20 minutes. Top chicken with low moisture mozzarella cheese and return to oven for 5 minutes.

Healthy Chicken Stacker
1 grilled chicken breast
2 tomato slices
1 lettuce leaf
1 slice of onion
1 slice of low moisture mozzarella cheese
2 slices of bacon, cooked
1 T mustard

Slice chicken breast in half to make breast half the width. On one half of breast place slice of mozzarella cheese and then bacon. Place in microwave approximately 30 seconds or until cheese is soft. On remaining half of breast spread mustard and add tomato, onion and lettuce leaf. Add each breast together to simulate a sandwich with breasts acting as the bread.

Hot Wings
24 skinless chicken wings
½ cup extra virgin olive oil
¼ cup vinegar
1 tsp. Tabasco sauce
1 tsp. garlic sauce
1 cup ranch dressing
Celery stalks

In a mixing bowl combine oil, vinegar, Tabasco sauce and garlic powder. Marinate wings in mixture for 1 hour. Preheat oven at 400 degrees. Coat large cookie sheet with organic olive oil. Arrange chicken wings on cookie sheet. Keep marinade aside. Bake wings for 20 minutes. Baste with marinade and broil for 10 minutes or until brown. Turn wings over, baste and broil another 10 minutes. Serve with celery and ranch dressing.

Lemon Caper Chicken

2 lbs. of boneless skinless chicken breasts
1 T extra virgin olive oil
½ cup white wine
1 T lemon juice
1 tsp. grated lemon zest
2 T capers, drained, rinsed
Sea salt and ground black pepper for desired taste

Place large skillet over medium heat until hot but not smoking. Sprinkle chicken with salt and pepper. Add chicken to skillet and cook until browned, 4 to 5 minutes per side. Remove chicken from skillet; cover and keep warm. Add wine, lemon juice, lemon zest and capers to same skillet. Bring to a boil, lower heat and simmer 2 minutes, scraping up any browned bits from bottom of skillet. Whisk in butter, 1 piece at a time, and cook over low heat until incorporated. Pour sauce over chicken and serve immediately.

Tasty Chicken Bake

4 boneless skinless chicken breasts
8 pieces of cooked bacon coarsely chopped
1 cup mushrooms, sliced
1 minced garlic clove
½ cup shredded low moisture mozzarella cheese
Seasonings of your choice

Add flavor to chicken with seasonings of your choice. Grill chicken until thoroughly cooked. Preheat oven to 350 degrees. Coat a medium sized skillet with organic olive oil cooking spray. Preheat over medium heat and sauté garlic and mushrooms. Coat a baking dish with organic olive oil. Place chicken breasts in baking dish. Top each breast with ¼ of bacon and mushrooms and then top with mozzarella cheese. Bake for 10 minutes.

Phase 3 – Fish & Seafood

Baked Salmon
1 lb. thawed salmon
2 tsp. garlic powder
1 T lemon juice
Sea salt and ground black pepper for desired taste

Preheat oven to 425 degrees. Coat baking dish with organic olive oil. Place salmon in baking dish. Sprinkle with garlic powder, lemon juice, sea salt and ground black pepper. Bake for 10-15 minutes. Baking times will depend on thickness of salmon. Bake until thickest part of salmon is thoroughly cooked.

Blackened Fish
4 fillets of preferred white fish
3 T paprika
1 tsp. sea salt
1 tsp. ground black pepper
1 T onion powder
1 tsp. thyme
1 tsp. oregano
1 tsp. basil
2 T grape seed oil
1 lemon juice
½ tsp. garlic powder

In a mixing bowl combine paprika, sea salt, ground black pepper, onion powder, thyme, oregano, and basil. Liberally coat both sides of fish. Allow fish to sit 10 minutes to absorb seasoning. Add grape seed oil to a large skillet. Preheat over medium heat. Once oils is almost smoking add fillets and cook 2-4 minutes on each side. Sprinkle with lemon juice.

Cod Topped with Artichokes and Crab

2 cod filets
1 can artichokes packed in water and drained
5 T grated mozzarella cheese
½ tsp. minced garlic
Sea salt and ground black pepper for desired taste

Preheat oven to 375 degrees. Spray glass baking dish with organic olive oil cooking spray. Place cod filets in dish. Coarsely chop 1 or 2 of the artichokes. In a small bowl, combine the chopped artichokes, crab, garlic and mozzarella cheese. Mix thoroughly. Season with sea salt and ground black pepper to taste. Spread mixture over top of the two filets. Cut remaining artichokes in half and place around the filets in the baking dish. Lightly sprinkle the top of the fish and artichokes with shredded mozzarella for a bit more browning. Bake for about 20-25 minutes or until fish is flakey and not dry.

Crab Cakes

1 lb. cooked Alaska king crab or snow crab
¼ cup onion, finely chopped
2 T mayonnaise
1 tsp. Dijon mustard
¼ cup egg whites
¼ cup pork rinds, finely crushed
1 T lemon juice
1/2 tsp. sea salt
1 ¼ tsp. Old Bay Seafood Spices

In a large mixing bowl combine all ingredients and mix well. Take the mixture and shape into 8 patties. Coat large skillet with organic olive oil and place over medium to high heat. Add the patties to the pan and cook for 3-4 minutes, then turn over and cook for another 3-4 minutes until golden brown.

Fried Tilapia
4 Tilapia filets
2 egg whites
¼ cup BBQ flavor pork rinds, finely crushed
Sea salt for desired taste

Beat egg whites with a fork until they become frothy. Spread pork rinds on flat plate. Coat medium skillet with organic olive oil. Preheat skillet over medium heat. Coat tilapia well with frothy egg whites. Pat pork rind crumbs thickly on both sides of tilapia. Carefully place tilapia in skillet. Fry on both sides until coating is slightly brown and fish is fully cooked.

Garlic Lobster Tails
4 medium sized lobster tails
2 minced garlic cloves
1 tsp. orange peel, finely shredded
¼ tsp. crushed red pepper
¼ tsp. cayenne pepper
3 T lemon juice

Preheat oven to broil. Butterfly the lobster tails by cutting through the hard top and meat of the tail. Spread the halves and place on broiler rack with the meat facing up. Coat small skillet with organic olive oil cooking spray. Preheat over medium heat. Add garlic, orange peel, cayenne pepper, crushed red pepper and lemon juice to skillet. Sauté for 3-5 minutes. Brush mixture over the lobster tails. Broil lobster tails 4 inches from heat about 15 minutes or until meat is opaque.

Mozzarella Mahi-Mahi

1 lb. Mahi-Mahi filets
4 T cottage cheese
4 tsp. grated Mozzarella cheese
2 tsp. Dijon mustard
2 tsp. lemon juice
2 tsp. fresh ground horseradish sauce
1 tsp. dill
1 tsp. parsley

Preheat oven to broil. Coat broiling pan with organic olive oil. Arrange fish on broiling pan. Combine the remaining ingredients in mixing bowl and mix thoroughly. Spread the sauce mixture over the filets in a thin layer. Place under broiler approximately 8 inches from heat for about 8 to 10 minutes or until fish flakes easily.

Mozzarella Salmon Fillet

1 lb. thawed salmon
1 tsp. garlic powder
2 T lemon juice
2 tsp. chives
½ cup mayonnaise
½ tsp. onion powder
¼ cup grated mozzarella cheese
Sea salt and ground pepper for desired taste

Preheat the oven to 400 degrees. In a small bowl combine all ingredients EXCEPT the salmon and mix well. Spread mayonnaise mix over the top of the salmon covering all of the meat. Coat baking dish with organic olive oil. Place salmon, skin side down, on a baking dish and cook for 25-30 minutes until the fish flakes with a fork and the topping is golden brown. Baking times will depend on thickness of salmon. Bake until thickest part of salmon is thoroughly cooked.

Mozzarella Scallops
1 lb. bay scallops
5 minced garlic cloves
2 tsp. extra virgin olive oil
1 10 oz. package of baby spinach
1 T basil
1 T parsley
2 large tomatoes, diced
1 tsp. ground black pepper
1 cup low moisture mozzarella cheese

In large skillet, sauté garlic in 1 tsp. of extra virgin olive oil over medium heat. Sauté till browned. Add spinach to skillet and sauté until soft. Remove spinach and drain in colander. Season scallops with basil and parsley. Add remaining tsp. of olive oil to skillet and sauté scallops. Add diced tomatoes and simmer 3 minutes. Stir spinach back into skillet until heated through. Add pepper and mozzarella cheese. Heat until cheese melts.

Roasted Halibut with Tomato and Cilantro
4 halibut fillets
2 T extra virgin olive oil
1 cup tomatoes, diced
1 tsp. ground black pepper
1 T shallots, chopped
3 T cilantro, chopped
2 tsp. minced garlic
3 T lime juice
1 tsp. sea salt
½ tsp. balsamic vinegar
¼ tsp. crushed red pepper

Preheat oven to 450°F. Coat a baking sheet with organic olive oil. Rub halibut with 2 teaspoons oil. Sprinkle halibut with pepper. Place halibut on the prepared baking sheet.

Transfer to the oven and roast until the fish flakes easily with a fork, 15 to 20 minutes, depending on the thickness of the fillet. Meanwhile, heat the remaining 1 teaspoon of extra virgin olive oil in a small skillet over medium heat. Add shallots and cook until they begin to soften, about 20 seconds. Add tomatoes and cook, stirring, until softened, about 1 ½ minutes. Stir in cilantro, minced garlic, sea salt, lime juice and vinegar. Simmer for 1 minute. Sir and remove from heat. Spoon the sauce over the halibut to serve.

Shrimp Scampi

½ lb. of shelled, de-veined, cooked shrimp
¼ tsp. garlic powder
1 tsp. lemon juice
½ tsp. parsley
Sea salt and ground pepper to desired taste

Coat a medium skillet with organic olive oil and preheat over medium heat. Add shrimp, garlic powder and lemon juice. Cook until watery liquid evaporates. Add sea salt and ground black pepper. Top with parsley.

Shrimp Skewers

16 peeled and de-veined jumbo shrimp
4 skewers
2 cloves garlic, minced
2 tbsp. extra virgin olive oil
2 tsp. chili powder
1 tsp. lemon zest
¼ cup freshly squeezed orange juice
¼ cup cilantro, finely chopped

Combine all ingredients in a large zip-lock bag. Coat shrimp evenly and marinate in refrigerator for 1 hour. Preheat grill to medium heat. Place on skewers, 4 shrimp per skewer. Grill over medium heat until pink approximately 2 minutes per side.

Shrimp Wrapped in Bacon

1 lb. raw, de-veined shrimp
½ lb. sugar free bacon
Toothpicks

Wrap ¼ slice of raw bacon around raw shrimp. Attach shrimp ends on inside curve of shrimp with toothpick. Insert toothpick all the way through the shrimp so it will lay flat to cook. Coat large skillet with organic olive oil. Preheat skillet over medium heat. Put wrapped shrimp in hot skillet. Fry until bacon is crispy.

Spiced Up Scallops

6 oz. extra-large scallops
½ tsp. paprika
½ tsp. ground black pepper
½ tsp. cayenne pepper
½ tsp. cumin
½ tsp. extra virgin olive oil
Dash of sea salt

Place dry scallops in mixing bowl and combine paprika, ground pepper, cumin and cayenne pepper. Mix well. Dredge each scallop in spice mixture and set aside. Heat olive oil in a small skillet until hot. Add scallops and sauté, about 3 minutes on each side, flipping once, or until cooked through. Sprinkle with the salt after cooking if desired.

Tuna Quiche

6 oz. canned tuna packed in water drained
¼ cup low moisture mozzarella cheese
3 T green onion, chopped
3 eggs
2 tbsp. heavy cream
½ tsp. dill
½ tsp. sea salt
Ground pepper for desired taste

Preheat oven to 350 degrees. Coat a pie plate with organic olive oil cooking spray. Add tuna, green onions, and cheese in pie plate. In mixing bowl beat the eggs, cream and seasonings till thoroughly mixed. Pour mixture into pie plate. Bake for 35 minutes.

Phase 3- Beef

Baked Meatballs
1 lb. ground beef
1 lb. Italian sausage
2 eggs
½ tsp. garlic powder
½ cup mozzarella cheese
½ tsp. sea salt
¼ tsp. ground black pepper

Preheat oven to 375 degrees. Combine all ingredients in a large mixing bowl. Thoroughly hand mix until meat no longer feels slimy from eggs. Shape into ping pong ball sized meatballs. Spray large baking sheet with organic olive oil. Place meatballs on baking sheet and bake 25 minutes or until cooked all the way through.

Barbecue Shredded Beef
2 lbs. chuck meat
3 cloves garlic
2 T chili powder
1 T vinegar
2 T oregano
2 T basil
1 T cumin
1 ½ cups sugar free barbecue sauce, set aside *(refer to recipe)*
1 ½ cups of bottled or filtered water
Add sea salt and ground black pepper to taste

Coat organic olive oil in a 4-6 quart soup pot over low heat. Cook beef till brown. Add all other ingredients, bring to boil. Cover and simmer for 1 ½ hours or longer until very tender. Uncover and boil until liquid almost evaporates. With 2 forks, shred meat. Add in barbeque sauce.

Barbecue Sloppy Joes

1 lb. organic grass feed beef
1 cup sugar free barbecue sauce *(refer to recipe)*
1 large onion, chopped
½ cup low moisture mozzarella cheese
6 large lettuce leaves

Wash lettuce leaves and place 2 leaves on 3 serving dishes. Spray organic olive oil on a small skillet and heat over medium heat. Add onion and sauté until tender. Set onions aside. Heat a large skillet over medium heat. Add beef and brown. Add Sugar free barbecue sauce and onions. Reduce heat and simmer for 10 minutes. Sprinkle mozzarella cheese on top. Serve on lettuce leaves.

Beefy Soft Taco

1 lb. of organic grass fed beef
8 T taco seasoning *(refer to recipe)*
6 large lettuce leaves
1 cup green pepper, chopped
1 large onion, chopped
¼ cup salsa *(refer to recipe)*
½ cup low moisture mozzarella cheese

Wash lettuce leaves and place 2 leaves on 3 serving dishes. In medium skillet brown the beef with taco seasoning. Half way through cooking add in green peppers and onion and continue to sauté until beef is fully cooked. Sprinkle mozzarella cheese on top and allow it to melt. Let cool a few minutes. Scoop beef mixture on to lettuce leaves. Top with salsa and wrap up leaves. Serve.

Beef Fajitas for the Whole Family

Marinade:

3 garlic cloves, pressed

1 tsp. sea salt

2 tsp. lime juice

1 jalapeno pepper, finely chopped

2 tsp. ground cumin

2 T olive oil

2 ½ lbs. sirloin steak

1 green bell pepper, cut in strips

1 red bell pepper, cut in strips

1 small red onion, sliced

1 cup salsa *(refer to recipe)*

¼ cup cilantro, chopped

2 T lime juice

6 cups lettuce, shredded

1 ¼ cup low moisture mozzarella cheese

Make Marinade: In a large bowl or re-sealable plastic bag, combine garlic, salt, lime juice, jalapeno, cumin and olive oil; whisk together. Add steak to marinade. Coat well. Marinate and refrigerate at least 1 hour. Remove steak from marinade. Discard marinade. Grill 3 to 4 minutes per side for medium-rare doneness and set aside. Coat large skillet with organic olive oil. Apply medium heat and add bell peppers, lime juice and onions and cook for 5 minutes, until vegetables are softened. Slice steak thinly across the grain. To assemble fajitas, place 1 cup of shredded lettuce on 6 serving plates. Place steak slices on top of lettuce and top with vegetable mix, salsa, mozzarella cheese and cilantro.

Breadless Cheesesteak

1 lb. grilled sirloin steak cut into strips
1 minced garlic clove
½ cup parsley
½ jalapeno, chopped
Dash of crushed red pepper flakes
1 ½ tsp. lime juice
¼ cup olive oil
¼ tsp. sea salt
1/8 tsp. ground black pepper
1 chopped red onion
2 large onions, chopped
3 cups lettuce, shredded
¾ cup shredded low moisture mozzarella cheese

Measure equal portions of lettuce onto 3 serving dishes. Place all ingredients EXCEPT steak, cheese, onion and tomatoes in a blender and blend until it is well combined. Pour into a mixing bowl and stir in the onions and tomatoes. Toss steak into mixture. Place mixture in a microwave safe dish and pour cheese on top. Microwave until cheese melts.

Chili

1 lb. organic grass feed beef
½ cup onions, chopped
¼ cup minced garlic
¼ cup green chili peppers, chopped
5 T organic tomato paste
¾ tsp. chili powder
½ tsp. cumin
¼ tsp. cayenne
¼ cup bottled or filtered water
1 packet Stevia

In a large skillet brown the ground beef with the onions and garlic. Mix in the bottle or filtered water, chili, peppers, tomato paste, chili powder, cumin, cayenne and Stevia. Stir thoroughly. Let simmer for 25- 30 minutes.

Crock Pot Roast

2 ½ lb. beef chuck roast
2 T extra virgin olive oil
4 cups of bottled or filtered water
8 minced garlic cloves
1 large onion, chopped
½ tsp. garlic salt
½ tsp. onion powder

Add extra virgin olive oil, onion powder and 1/4 tsp. garlic salt to a large skillet pan and heat. Sear beef on all sides. Put bottled or filtered water and remaining garlic salt into crock pot and turn crock pot to low heat. Place beef and flavored oil from skillet into the crock pot and cook on low for 6-8 hours. Add onion and garlic during the last hour of cooking. If you add them earlier, they will absorb the salts and the meat won't have as much flavor.

Garden Beef Bake

1 lb. organic grass fed beef
½ cup onion, chopped
1 ½ cups no meat tomato sauce *(refer to recipe)*
1 ¼ cup mozzarella cheese
1 med zucchini, sliced
½ cup mushrooms, sliced
½ tsp. oregano, basil, salt
½ tsp. basil
½ tsp. sea salt

Preheat oven to 350 degrees. Coat organic olive oil in a skillet and cook zucchini, onion and mushrooms until tender. Brown ground beef in pan and add tomato sauce with seasonings. Coat organic olive oil in a baking dish. Mix beef with vegetables and put in baking dish. Top with cheese. Bake uncovered at 350 for 30 min.

Hamburger Florentine

2 lbs. organic grass feed beef
1 10 oz. bag of spinach, thawed, drained, chopped
1 cup mushrooms, sliced
1 T minced garlic
½ cup onions, chopped
½ cup grated mozzarella cheese
2 tbsp. heavy cream
1 tsp. sea salt
½ tsp. ground black pepper

Preheat oven to 350 degrees. Coat a 2 quart casserole dish with organic olive oil. In a large skillet brown the beef and onion. Drain excess fat. Stir in spinach and mix until it well combined. Stir in sea salt, ground black pepper, minced garlic and mushrooms and stir until blended. Mix in mozzarella, cream, and mix well. Pour mixture into casserole dish and bake uncovered for 35 minutes or until bubbly and browned.

Meatloaf
1 lb. organic grass feed beef
1 lb. bulk Italian pork sausage
¾ cup onion, chopped
2 eggs
1 ½ tsp. dry mustard
½ tsp. sea salt
½ tsp. ground black pepper
1 ¼ cup pork rinds, finely crushed
¼ tsp. garlic powder
1 cup no meat tomato sauce *(refer to recipe)*

Preheat oven to 350 degrees. In a large mixing bowl combine the ground beef, bulk sausage, onion, eggs and mix thoroughly. Add the dry mustard, salt, pepper, dry breadcrumbs, garlic powder and ½ cup tomato sauce. Set aside remaining half cup of sauce. Mix ingredients thoroughly. Shape the meat into a loaf and place in a 9x5 baking pan. Pour the remaining tomato sauce over the top. Bake for 1 hour and 15 minutes or until the meat loaf is done.

Mushroom Bacon Cheeseburgers
1 lb. organic grass fed beef grilled into four patties
4 bacon slices
½ lb. mushrooms, sliced
½ cup onions, chopped
1tsp minced garlic
4 mozzarella cheese slices

Combine bacon, mushrooms, onions and minced garlic in a large skillet. Cook until all contents are brown. Drain excess fat. Top beef patties with mixture. Then top with cheese.

Oven Barbecued Beef

3 lb. beef brisket or rump roast
2 cups no sugar added barbeque sauce *(refer to recipe)*
1 large onion, chopped
2 minced garlic cloves
¾ cup of bottled or filtered water

Marinate beef in no sugar added barbecue sauce over night in refrigerator. Preheat oven to 350 degrees. Place beef in roasting pan. Pour remaining sauce on top of beef. Add onions and minced garlic. Gently add bottled or filtered water to bottom of baking dish. Cover with tin foil and bake for 3- 3 ½ hours.

Pizza Burger

1 lb. organic grass feed beef
½ tsp. sea salt
½ no meat tomato sauce *(refer to recipe)*
4 slices of low moisture mozzarella cheese

Combine beef, salt and no meat tomato sauce in a mixing bowl. Mold into 4 patties and pan-fry on a skillet over medium heat for 5-6 minutes on each side. Just before burgers are done, top each with spoonful pizza of sauce and 1 slice of low moisture mozzarella cheese.

Bacon Cheeseburgers
2 lbs. of organic grass feed beef
8 slices of chopped cooked bacon
½ cup shredded mozzarella cheese
½ cup scallions, chopped
½ tsp. sea salt
½ tsp. ground black pepper
¼ tsp. garlic powder
Sliced mozzarella cheese is optional

In a large mixing bowl combine all ingredients and thoroughly hand mix. Shape into 6 patties and grill. Top with a slice of cheese if desired.

Chapter 7

Phase 4 - The Rest of Your Life

Once you have reached your desired goal weight and followed the 3 week Phase 3 maintenance, you will continue to Phase 4, which you will follow for the rest of your life. Sugars and starches are slowly added into your diet in Phase 4. Eat breakfast like a king; eat lunch like a queen; eat dinner like a pauper. Load your calories earlier in the day. Late day eating is very hard on your metabolism and encourages weight gain. A minimum of 9 months of being absolutely vigilant about staying within 2 pounds +/- of your stabilized weight is a necessity. There are many cases where dieters will re-gain the weight lost by jumping back into their old eating habits. You can correct a splurge by simply utilizing phase 3 clean eating for a few days. It is important to understand that you cannot go back to your old ways without going back to your old body.

Continue to take your Supplements as recommended. Limit one starchy carbohydrate per day if possible.

- Try to eat healthy whole grains, multi-grains, or wheat pastas and breads.
- Use brown rice not white.
- Try sweet potatoes in place of white potatoes.
- Avoid using white flour starch when cooking as much as possible.
- Avoid fried foods and fast foods.

- Read food labels so you know what you are buying. Avoid anything with corn syrup solids or high fructose corn syrup which is a major factor in weight gain.

- Use Stevia as a sweetener. It is a natural product and does not have the same metabolic effects of the artificial sweeteners which can add to your weight gain and trigger sugar cravings.

- Know the caloric values of your alcoholic beverages. They are not forbidden but there are ~~lots~~ a lot of calories in a mixed drink (125 calories per ounce of hard spirit plus the calories of the mixer).

- Always eat breakfast in the morning. Do not skip that meal. Use a meal replacement if you are not into cooking or find yourself in a rush to get out the door.

- Eat your carbs earlier in the day. It is easier on your metabolism and does not encourage late-eating weight gain.

- Do not eat within 3 hours of bedtime. It encourages weight gain and encourages acid reflux.

- When you buy groceries, do the majority of your shopping around the outer perimeter of the store. The fresh fruits, veggies, dairy, and meats are stored there. Down the aisles are all the processed foods that are not so good for you.

- If you cannot manage fresh vegetables, buy frozen ones. Do not buy canned.

- Take your supplements. Under the supervision of your health care provider, increase the status of your health by taking omega 3 supplements, fish oils, CoQ10, antioxidants, etc. All of these add to your health.

- Never allow more than 1 starchy carbohydrate on your plate with each meal.

- Limit your sweets intake to special occasions and increase your exercise regimen the following day.

- Allow yourself a "cheat day" once a week and indulge in <u>one meal</u> at your favorite restaurant.

- Avoid foods that have a high glycemic load. Note: This is not the same as the glycemic index.

- Drink at least 2-3 quarts of water daily.

- Exercise is critical to weight maintenance; no getting around this fact.

You may integrate starches into your diet but choose wheat pasta, whole grain breads, sweet potatoes, multi-grain cereals and limit your refined sugars. Try to exercise at least 3 times per week, take your daily vitamins and supplements, and drink plenty of water. It is recommended to incorporate starches into your diet slowly by allowing only 1 starch daily for a week in Phase 4 and then increasing to 2 as desired thereafter. Some people are sensitive to wheat products and for those folks, wheat is a major source of inflammation and weight gain.

Avoid Trans Fats

Trans fat is a common name for unsaturated fat. Trans fats do not exist in nature but are made during a process called Hydrogenation for the purpose of food production. During this process, liquid vegetable oil is heated and combined with hydrogen gas. Partially hydrogenating vegetable oils make them more stable and less likely to spoil, which is very good for food manufacturers and very bad for you.

No amount of trans fats is healthy. The consumption of trans fats increases the risk of coronary heart disease by raising levels of "bad" LDL cholesterol and lowering levels of "good" HDL cholesterol.

Sources of Trans Fats

The major source of trans fats in the Western diet comes from commercially-prepared baked goods and snack foods:

- **Baked goods** – cookies, crackers, cakes, muffins, pie crusts, pizza dough, and some breads like hamburger buns
- **Fried foods** – doughnuts, French fries, fried chicken, chicken nuggets, and hard taco shells
- **Snack foods** – potato, corn, and tortilla chips; candy; packaged or microwave popcorn
- **Solid fats** – stick margarine and semi-solid vegetable shortening
- **Pre-mixed products** – cake mix, pancake mix, and chocolate drink mix

Calculating Daily Caloric Intake for PHASE 4

Maintenance

When you have reached your desired goal weight, and after successfully completing the maintenance interval, you continue onto Phase 4, which will be followed for the rest of your life. Sugars and starches are slowly added into your diet in Phase 4. Those starches consist of healthy whole grain or wheat pasta and bread, brown rice and sweet potatoes. Avoid white flour starches as much as possible. Try to limit yourself to one starch serving daily.

Step 1

Calculate your daily calorie intake with the following equation: Active males can determine the number of calories needed to maintain body weight by multiplying their weight in pounds by 15, while active females should multiply their weight by 12. Inactive males should calculate daily caloric intake by multiplying their body weight by 13, and inactive females should multiply their weight by 10.

Example: Male 175 x 13 = 2275 daily calories
Female 140 x 12 = 1680 daily calories

Step 2

Determine how many of your calories should be derived from fat by using the number of calories determined through the first equation and multiply the number by 30, or 30 percent for the number of fat calories you need daily.

Example: Male 2275 x .30 = 682.50 fat calories/day
Female 1680 x .30 = 504 fat calories/day

Step 3

Figure the number of grams that constitute the number of fat calories needed each day to maintain body weight by dividing the number of fat calories by nine. The resulting number is the amount of fat grams you should take in daily.

Example: Male 682.50/9 = 75.83 fat grams/day
Female 504/9 = 56 fat grams/day

Step 4

Lose one pound per week by creating a calorie deficit of 500 calories daily. For example, if your body requires 2,000 calories to maintain your body weight, you should take in only 1,500 calories per day to lose a steady pound per week. Gain one pound per week by adding an additional 500 calories to your determined daily calorie intake. Then re-calculate your fat calories and fat grams.

Phase 4 FOOD CHOICES

Proteins	Protein Grams	Carb Grams	Fat Grams	Calories	Sodium Mg
Chicken (no skin)	27	0	2	133	57
Turkey	28	0	2	132	58
Tuna (white canned in water)	30	0	1	140	127
Tuna (blue fin)	28	0	5	165	0
Beef (95% lean)	25	0	5	153	73
Tofu (firm)	18	4	9	164	16
Lobster	19	0.5	2	103	0
Shrimp	21	2	1	103	0
Crab	20	0	2	105	0
Scallops	17	4	0	92	289
Swordfish	22	0	5	134	0
Egg whites (4)	14	1	1	68	220
Whey Protein (1)	16	1	1	78	40
Cottage Cheese 1%	14	4	1	90	350

*4 oz. portions unless specified.

Starch	Protein Grams	Carb Grams	Fat Grams	Calories	Sodium Mg
Brown Rice	2	22	0.5	103	2.5
White Rice	2	23	0	103	1.5
Oatmeal	5	23	3	132	2
Cream of Rice Cereal	2	24	0	105	0
Popcorn (air)	3	22	1.5	109	4
Sweet Potato (4 oz.)	2	30	0	130	11
White Potato (4 oz.)	2	20	0	86	4
Corn (4 oz.)	3.5	22	0.5	93	1
Peas (4 oz.)	6	15	0	83	146
Multigrain Bread (sl)	2.5	18	1	00	170
Wheat Shredded	3	23	0	83	1

*1 oz. portions unless specified.

	Protein Grams	Carb Grams	Fat Grams	Calories	Sodium Mg
Fruits					
Banana (1 Med.)	0.9	18.5	0.3	72	0.8
Apple (1 Small)	0.3	14.6	0.2	55	1.1
Grapes (1 Cup)	1.2	29	0.3	110	3.2
Strawberries (1 Cup)	1	11.1	0.5	46	1.5
Orange (1 Small)	0.9	11.3	0.1	45	0
Melon (1 Small)	1.3	12.7	0.3	53	25
Pear (1 Small)	0.5	21.5	0.2	81	1.5
Grapefruit (1 Small)	0.6	8.1	0.1	32	0
Blackberries (1 Cup)	2	13.8	0.7	62	1.4
Blueberries (1 Cup)	1.1	21	0.5	83	1.5
Peaches (1 Cup)	1.5	16.2	0.4	66	0
Kiwi (1 Med.)	0.9	11.1	0.4	46	2.3
Cherries (1 Cup w/out pits)	1.2	18.7	0.2	74	0
Pineapple (1 Cup)	0.8	19.6	0.2	74	1.6

	Protein Grams	Carb Grams	Fat Grams	Calories	Sodium Mg
Vegetables					
Green Beans	3	10	0	44	2
Broccoli	5	9	0	50	29
Asparagus	6	7	1	40	3
Carrots	2	16	0	71	80
Mushrooms	4	8	0	48	25
Peppers, green	2	8	0	38	22
Romaine (2 cups)	2	3	0	16	0
Celery	0	8	0	29	214
Cucumbers	1	6	0	26	10
Cauliflower	4	8	0	46	22
Spinach	5	6	0	40	97
Iceberg Lettuce	1	5	0	22	15
Cabbage	2	9	0	40	34
Tomatoes	2	8	0	37	5

6 oz. portions unless specified.

171

What is the Glycemic Index?

Not all carbohydrate foods are created equal: in fact they behave quite differently in our bodies. The glycemic index (GI) describes this difference by ranking carbohydrates according to their effect on our blood glucose levels. Eating a lot of high GI foods can be detrimental to your health because it pushes your body to extremes. This is especially true if you are overweight and sedentary. Switch to eating mainly low GI carbs (the ones that produce only small fluctuations in our blood glucose and insulin levels) is the secret to long-term health; thus reducing your risk of heart disease and diabetes which is the key to sustainable weight-loss.

- Low GI means a smaller rise in blood glucose levels after meals
- Low GI diets can help people lose weight
- Low GI diets can improve the body's sensitivity to insulin
- High GI foods help re-fuel carbohydrate levels after exercise
- Low GI can improve diabetes control
- Low GI foods keep you fuller for longer

What is the Glycemic Load?

The glycemic index compares the potential of foods containing the same amount of carbohydrate to raise blood glucose. However, the amount of carbohydrate consumed also affects blood glucose levels and insulin responses. The **glycemic load** of a food is calculated by multiplying the glycemic index by the amount of carbohydrate in grams provided by a food and dividing the total by 100. Dietary glycemic load is the sum of the glycemic loads for all foods consumed in the diet. The concept of glycemic load was developed by scientists to simultaneously describe the quality (glycemic index) and quantity of carbohydrate in a meal or diet.

- Glycemic load builds on the GI to provide a measure of total glycemic response to a food or meal
- Glycemic load = GI (%) x grams of carbohydrate per serving and dividing the total by 100
- One unit of GL ~ glycemic effect of 1 gram glucose
- You can sum the GL of all the foods in a meal, for the whole day or even longer
- A typical diet has ~ 100 GL units per day (range 60 - 180)
- The GI database gives both GI & GL values

In the first two hours after a meal, blood glucose and insulin levels rise higher after a high-glycemic load meal than they do after a low-glycemic load meal containing equal calories. However, in response to the excess insulin secretion, blood glucose levels drop lower over the next few hours after a high-glycemic load meal than they do after a low-glycemic load meal. This may explain why 15 out of 16 published studies found that the consumption of low-glycemic index foods delayed the return of hunger, decreased subsequent food intake, and increased satiety (feeling full) when compared to high-glycemic index foods. The results of several small short-term trials (1-4 months) suggest that low-glycemic load diets result in significantly more weight or fat loss than high-glycemic load diets. Although long-term randomized controlled trials of low-glycemic load diets in the treatment of obesity are lacking, the results of short-term studies on appetite regulation and weight-loss suggest that low glycemic-load diets may be useful in promoting long-term weight-loss and decreasing the prevalence of obesity and Type 2 Diabetes.

Low-Glycemic Index Foods

Less Than 55

Artichoke	15
Asparagus	15
Broccoli	15
Cauliflower	15
Celery	15
Cucumber	15
Eggplant	15
Green beans	15
Lettuce, all varieties	15
Peppers, all varieties	15
Snow peas	15
Spinach	15
Young summer squash	15
Zucchini	15
Tomatoes	15

Cherries	22
Peas, dried	22
Plum	24
Grapefruit	25
Pearled barley	25
Peach	28
Canned peaches, natural juice	30
Dried apricots	31
Soy milk	30
Baby lima beans, frozen	32
Fat-free milk	32
Fettuccine	32
M&M's Chocolate Candies, Peanut	32
Low-fat yogurt, sugar sweetened	33
Apple	36
Pear	36
Whole wheat spaghetti	37
Tomato soup	38
Carrots, cooked	39

Mars Snickers Bar	40
Apple juice	41
Spaghetti	41
All-Bran	42
Canned chickpeas	42
Custard	43
Grapes	43
Orange	43
Canned lentil soup	44
Canned pinto beans	45
Macaroni	45
Pineapple juice	46
Banana bread	47
Long-grain rice	47
Parboiled rice	47
Bulgur	48
Canned baked beans	48
Grapefruit juice	48
Green peas	48

Oat bran bread	48
Chocolate bar, 1.5 oz	49
Old-fashioned oatmeal	49
Cheese tortellini	50
Low-fat ice cream	50
Canned kidney beans	52
Kiwifruit	52
Orange juice, not from concentrate	52
Banana	53
Potato chips	54
Pound cake	54
Special K	54
Sweet potato	54

Tips on Eating Out

Fast food restaurants are an easy and defeating solution. Fast food is packed with exactly what humans are genetically programmed to desire: sugar and fat! In fact, ketchup, one of America's favorite condiments, is simply a sweet way to deliver the salt and fat found in French fries. Most fast foods have a high calorie count and high glycemic carbohydrates, leading to an enormous amount of calories and too little satiety. You can find meals that are low in saturated fat, *trans* fat, and cholesterol in any restaurant by simply making a special request to the chef.

Don't be shy about making special requests; most restaurants will probably honor your request. Ask your server if the "catch of the day" such as orange roughy has been pre-marinated in a butter or herb sauce, if the answer is NO, then ask to have it grilled or broiled plain with lemon.

➢ When ordering vegetables, make sure they are steamed without butter and have no seasonings added which could contain very high amounts of sodium.

➢ A rule of thumb, always ask to have any condiment on the side, this way YOU will be in control of how much flavor, fat and salt you are going to consume, if at all.

➢ Bring your salad dressing with you to the restaurant. Most restaurants have oil & vinegar or vinaigrette if you forget.

➢ Ask your server if the kitchen can alter preparations to meet your needs, or call ahead before you choose your restaurant. If your food isn't prepared as you requested, send it back.

For example, some individuals think that 3 ounces of chicken is any piece of a full chicken, when in actuality it is the size of a deck of cards or the palm of your hand. 1 cup of fruits or vegetables equals the size of a baseball and a medium potato equals the size of a computer mouse. Once you can approximate the calories of a portion of food by looking at it, you may want to discontinue weighing and measuring food.

Dining Ideas

1. Portion size is important. Help control your weight by asking for smaller portions, sharing entrees with a companion, or putting half of your meal in a to-go box to enjoy another time.

2. Skip parts of the meal you like less. Have an "I can eat that food any old time" approach.

3. Go to places where you can order healthy, low fat meals.

4. Ask to substitute high fat items like French fries for a baked potato or side salad instead.

5. Eat a little less for lunch to save for a special dinner later, but don't skip meals. This can lead to over eating.

6. Eat a snack at least 30 minutes before your meal to help be in better control of your choices. Try a piece of fruit like an apple or have a glass of water with lemon.

7. Avoid buffets and all-you-can-eat specials.

8. Order an appetizer as a main course instead.

9. Alcoholic beverages can stimulate your appetite. Plus, there are almost 200 calories per ounce which can add up fast. Remember overall calories are just as important as watching fat and carbohydrate content.

10. When dining out, remember this: The menu doesn't necessarily tell you what your food choices are, it tells you what ingredients the chef has in the kitchen to work with. Many restaurants will customize a meal for you if you ask them to.

Eating Healthy During the Holiday Season

For many people, holidays and family get-togethers are a time for celebration. These celebrations often involve foods that are high in fat, sugar and calories and short on nutrition. With a few minor changes, however, special occasion foods can be both delicious and nutritious.

- Avoid fast food. The holiday season can keep you on the go with little time to prepare meals. Fast food may be handy, but often is high in fat. Prepare and freeze quick, healthy meals ahead of time to stay out of the fast food trap.

- Don't go to a party starving. Before you leave home, eat something light or drink a meal replacement shake. Also drink a great deal of water the day of the party.

- Alcoholic beverages can pack on the calories, so if you're drinking alcohol, choose a light beer or a champagne spritzer. Watch out for the Egg Nog - it is high in calories and fat.

- Offer to bring a low-calorie dish to holiday parties. Your host might appreciate it, and you'll know that at least one healthy item will be on hand.

- If you are at the mercy of the dinner host, eat modest amounts of the foods offered and fill up on foods with more fiber and volume and fewer calories. Make a small plate and skip the seconds.

- Just because it is the holidays doesn't mean you should give yourself the license to eat everything that passes by. Factor in the little extras into your daily intake.

- If you are staying with family or friends ask them if you can have a space in the refrigerator and keep foods on hand to snack on like lean deli meats, cottage cheese, nonfat cheese sticks, etc.

- Most people have a little extra time available over the holiday season when they are not at work. Take this opportunity to develop a regular exercise regimen. This will help to burn off the excess calories and fat consumed over this period. It will also get you into the habit of exercising, and you can continue the regimen after the holiday season is over.

Chapter 8

Exercise Routine

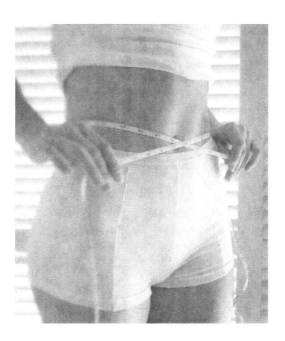

Exercise is a crucial part to your weight loss and overall health!

It is recommended that you exercise or engage in your favorite physical activity at least 3 times per week.

EXERCISE PROGRAMS SHOULD NOT BE STARTED WITHOUT SEEKING YOUR PHYSICIAN'S APPROVAL!

Why Should You Stretch?

The Benefits

Stretching is an important part of a cool down, not only physically but mentally. Finishing your workout feeling good can help you associate those good feelings with future workouts. Other benefits include:

- Improving your performance and reducing your risk of injury
- Reducing muscle soreness and improving your posture
- Helping reduce lower back pain
- Increasing blood and nutrients to the tissues
- Improving your coordination
- Enjoying your exercise more and helping reduce stress

The Basics

Your stretching program doesn't have to be complicated. Following these simple rules can make your routine safe and easy:

- Make sure you stretch warm muscles. Stretching cold muscles can cause injuries, so save the stretching for after your workout.
- Never bounce when you stretch. This forces the muscle to go beyond what is comfortable and can cause injury.
- Stretch all the muscles you use during your workout, focusing on any areas that are tight or tender.
- Hold each stretch for about 15-30 seconds and try to do each stretch 2 or more times.

Stretching and flexibility programs have become so popular, it's easy to learn how to do it safely and there are a number of tools out there to make your routine a little more effective. Skipping stretching will invite injury and lengthen your recovery time.

Most Common Cardio Exercises

You already know that one of the most important things you can do for your weight loss goals is regular cardio exercise. There are so many choices out there...which exercises are the most effective? Below are the best cardio activities for burning calories and getting in great shape.

Running

Running is one of best activities you can do. It doesn't require special equipment (except some quality shoes) and you can do it anywhere. Best of all, you burn serious calories, especially if you add hills and sprints. A 145-lb person can burn 300 calories (at 5.2 mph) in 30 minutes. The downside is that it takes a lot of practice and you should watch your knees and ankles for any discomfort or pain.

Walking

Walking is a great exercise, burning about 180 calories in 30 minutes. Adding hills, sprints or even a few minutes of jogging can increase the amount of calories you burn. Make sure you walk briskly; imagine you are trying to catch a bus, while keeping your head up, back straight, and swinging your arms. Try to walk at an incline on a treadmill because it will burn more calories.

Bicycling

Outdoors or indoors, cycling gives some great cardio. Using all the power in your legs, you'll increase endurance while burning a lot of calories; anywhere from 250-500 in 30 minutes, depending on how fast you go and how high your resistance is.

Elliptical Trainer

The elliptical trainer is a great way to build endurance while protecting your aching joints from high impact activities. Plus, if you use one with arms, it's just like using a cross-country ski machine. The elliptical trainer is also a good choice for runners looking for a break from pounding the pavement. A 145 lb. person burns about 300 calories in 30 minutes.

Swimming

Swimming, like cross-country skiing, is a full body exercise. The more body parts you involve in your workout, the more calories you'll burn. Spend 30 minutes doing the breast stroke and you'll burn almost 400 calories. Best of all, your joints are fully supported so you don't have to worry about high-impact injuries. It's also great cross-training for other cardio activities.

Step Aerobics

Step aerobics has yet to lose its luster for many gym-goers and it's a good thing. Step is one tough workout that targets your legs, buttocks and hips while burning almost 400 calories in 30 minutes (during high intensity sessions). Though it might be complicated, step is easy to learn if you start with a beginner class or video.

Weight Loss: Your Health & Safety

People who are overweight or obese increase their risk for developing heart disease, diabetes, some forms of cancer, gall bladder disease, osteoarthritis, and sleep apnea. Losing even small amounts of weight (five to ten percent of body weight), may reduce these risks. The side effects and complications some people may experience while losing weight by following a healthy eating plan and exercise program are usually minor compared to the risks involved with being overweight or obese.

Children, adolescents, pregnant or breast feeding women, and people with significant health problems such as heart disease, breast cancer, prostate cancer or any type of cancer, kidney disease, liver disease, or uncontrolled diabetes should not begin this program without close supervision by their primary care provider.

Dieters under treatment for other conditions or taking medications prescribed by their health care provider should inform their providers before beginning this diet because, in some cases, adjustments to medications or modifications to the weight loss program may be appropriate.

It is my desire that the updated information and tools you have obtained within this book-will enable you to follow a safer and more comfortable dieting experience that delivers the same results as the original. Sometimes results are even better!

Appendix

Article References

"Fighting America's Obesity Epidemic"; SOURCE; *The San Diego Union Tribune;* Morton Kondracke; April 17th 2005; *www.signonsandiego.com/uniontrib/20050417/ news_mz1e17morton.html*

"The Truth about Fad Diets"; SOURCE: Nielsen, ST; Popkins; *Journal of the American Medical Association* 2003; Vol. 28p (4): pp 450-453; *www.webmd.com/diet/the-truth-about-fad-diets*

"Apple Cider Vinegar"; Web MD Medical Reference; SOURCES: Hill, L. *Journal of the American Dietetic Association*, July 2005; vol 105: pp 1141-1144; *Medscape General Medicine*, 2006; vol 8. Korkmaz, A. *Pediatric Dermatology*, January/February, 2000; vol 17: pp 34-36. Ostman, E. *European Journal of Clinical Nutrition*, 2005; vol. 59: pp 983-88. Social Issues Research Centre web site: "1958." University of Texas M.D. Andersen Cancer Center: "Complementary/Integrative Medicine Therapies: Apple Cider Vinegar." White, A. *Diabetes Care*, November 2007; vol 30: pp 2814-15. *www.webmd.com/diet/apple-cider-vinegar?page2=*

"Leptin Resistance and Obesity". 2007; 16(1): 50-57; SOURCE; http://www.scopemed.org/?mno=19794

"Weight loss: 6 strategies for success"; SOURCE: Dec. 20, 2006; 1998-2008 Mayo Foundation for Medical Education and Research (MFMER), *http://mayoclinic.com/health/ weight-loss/HQ01625*

"Obesity, Weight loss, and Very Low Calorie Diets (VLCD's)"; SOURCE: WebMD Medical Reference provided in collaboration with the Cleveland Clinic; Reviewed by Jonathan L. Gelfand, MD on February 11, 2008; Edited by Cynthia Dennison Haines, MD on October 1, 2005; *http://www.webmd.com/diet/low-calorie-diets*

"Coconut Oil: Why it is good for you?" SOURCE: authored by Dr. Lita Lee; *www.coconutoil.com/litalee.htm*

"Calorie restriction and aging: a review of the literature and implications for studies in humans;" SOURCE; *American Journal of Clinical Nutrition* (2003; volume 78, pp 361–69) by Leonie K. Heilbronn and Eric Ravussin who are renowned and respected scientists.

"How to Cleanse and Detoxify Your Body Today!", SOURCE: authored by: Elson M. Haas, MD

"Healthy Weight – What affects your weight?" SOURCE; WebMD medical reference; *Healthwise, Incorporated* © 1995-2008; recent update May 25th, 2007; Authored by: Caroline Rea RN, BSN, MS and Jeaneatte Curtis; *http://www.webmd.com/diet/tc/healthy-weight-what-affects-your-weight*

"Why diets should be history"; Cro-Magnon Lesson: *We're Fat Because We're Starving!* authored by: David Zinczenko; editor in chief of *Men's Health* and author of the new book, "The Abs Diet"; *USA Today* Reprint; "THE FORUM"© Copyright 2004 *USA TODAY*, a division of Ganneti Co. Inc.

"Consumption of high-fructose corn syrup in beverages may play a role in the epidemic of obesity;" SOURCE: *The American Journal of Clinical Nutrition;* authored by: George A. Bray, Samara Joy Nielsen and Barry M. Popkin;

Vol. 79, No. 4, pp 537-543; April 2004; © 2004 American Society for Clinical Nutrition

"Colas, but not other carbonated beverages, are associated with low bone mineral density in older women: The Framingham Osteoporosis Study; SOURCE: *The American Journal of Clinical Nutrition;* authored by: Katherine L. Tucker, Kyoko Morita, Ning Qiao, Marian T. Hannan, L. Adrienne Cupples and Douglas P. Kie; Vol. 84, No. 4, 936-942; October 2006; © 2006 American Society for Nutrition

"High-fiber foods boost health" and help control your weight;" SOURCE; *www.webmd.com* authored by: By Elaine Magee, MPH, RD; reviewed by: Brunilda Nazario, MD

"Grapefruit and Weight Loss;" SOURCE: *http://www.medicalnewstoday.com/articles/5495.php;* referred by: Nutrition and Metabolic Research Center at Scripps; January 24, 2004

"UNC researchers find MSG use linked to obesity;" SOURCE: Liancheng Zhao from University of North Carolina Research Dept. and researchers from the Cardiovascular Institute at the Chinese Academy of Medical Sciences in Beijing; August 13, 2008 *http://www.nature.com/oby/journal/v16/n8/full/oby2008274a.htm (clinical study)*

"High Blood Pressure;" SOURCE: *The Merck Manuals, Online Medical Library*; authored by: George L. Bakris MD; Last full review/revision April 2007 *http://www.merck.com/mmhe/sec03/ch022/ch022a.html*

References

"Successful Weight Loss Intervention Using a Modified hCG Diet"; SOURCE; *The Bariatrician;* December 2010

http://www.weightshop.net/documents/Bryman%20HCG%20Article.pdf

"Chorionic Gonadotropin in Obesity: Further Clinical Observations," authored by: Harry A. Gusman, M.D.; SOURCE; *The American Journal of Clinical Nutrition*

"Effects of human chorionic gonadotropin on weight loss, hunger, and feeling of well being," authored by: W.L. Asher, M.D. and Harold W. Harper M.D.; SOURCE; *The American Journal of Clinical Nutrition*

Simeons, Dr. ATW, 1954. HCG Diet Manuscript by Dr. ATW Simeons - "Pounds and Inches"; Rome, Italy

Extreme Weight Loss - The Definitive HCG Protocol for Vegans and Vegetarians; authored by: Rebekah Sue Niman; paperback 2012

Suzanne Somers Slim and Sexy Forever: The Hormone Solution for Permanent Weight Loss and Optimal Living; authored by: Suzanne Somers; paperback April 25, 2006

License, Disclaimers and Terms of Use Agreement

IMPORTANT: Read the following terms and conditions and disclaimers carefully before using applying any weight loss program. Using this free document indicates your acceptance of these terms and conditions. If you do not agree with these terms and conditions, promptly return the document to HCG Doctors Group, LLC.

This document is a license agreement ("License Agreement") between you, an individual or business ("Licensee" or "You"), and HCG Doctors Group, LLC and any other company directly associated with HCG Doctors Group, LLC in any form or business function. As used in this License Agreement, the term "SOFTWARE" means any software that may be included on a CD or accessed through the Internet. The term "SOFTWARE" does not include any software that is covered by a separate license offered or granted by a person other than HCG Doctors Group, LLC. The SOFTWARE and accompanying documentation ("Documentation") and any copies or modifications are referenced together as the "Licensed Product."

1. PROPRIETARY RIGHTS. The Licensed Product and the procedures listed within this book are the proprietary products of HCG Doctors Group, LLC or its licensors and is protected under Federal copyright laws and international treaty provisions. Ownership of the Licensed Product and all copies, modifications, translations, copyrights, trademarks, patents and specialized procedures thereof shall at all times remain with HCG Doctors Group, LLC or its licensors.

2. GRANT OF LICENSE. The Licensed Product is being licensed to you, which means you have the right to use the Licensed Product only in accordance with this License Agreement. The SOFTWARE is considered in use on a computer when it is loaded into temporary memory or installed into permanent memory or accessed by the Internet.

3. PERSONAL LICENSE. This license is personal to you. You may not sublicense, lease, sell, or otherwise transfer the Licensed Product to any other person. You may use the Licensed Product only for your own personal use if you are an individual or for your own internal business purposes if you are a business. Notwithstanding the foregoing, the

Licensed Product shall not be used to process information of any other entity as a service bureau.

4. HUMAN CHORIONIC GONADOTROPIN. Human Chorionic Gonadotropin ("HCG") is a hormone found in the urine of pregnant women. More than 50 years ago, Dr. Albert T. Simeons, a British-born physician, contended that HCG injections would enable dieters to subsist comfortably on a 500-calorie-a-day diet. He claimed that HCG would mobilize stored fat; suppress appetite; and redistribute fat from the waist, hips and thighs. There is no scientific evidence to support these claims. Moreover, a 500-calorie (semi-starvation) diet is likely to result in loss of protein from vital organs, and HCG can cause other adverse effects. Gabe Mirkin, MD has noted that at one time HCG was the most widespread obesity medication administered in the United States; however, additional independent research showed that HCG alone does not cause weight loss and is only a small portion of a total weight loss management program.

5. GOVERNMENT REGULATION/HCG REQUIRED DISCLAIMERS. In 1976, the Federal Trade Commission ordered the Simeon Management Corporation, Simeon Weight Clinics Foundation, Bariatrics Management Corporation, C.M. Norcal, Inc., HCG Weight Clinics Foundation and their officers to stop claiming that their HCG-based programs were safe, effective and/or approved by the Food and Drug Administration for weight-control. Although the order did not stop the clinics from using HCG, it required that patients who contract for the treatment be informed in writing that:

THESE WEIGHT REDUCTION TREATMENTS INCLUDE THE INJECTION OF HCG, A DRUG WHICH HAS NOT BEEN APPROVED BY THE FOOD AND DRUG ADMINISTRATION AS SAFE AND EFFECTIVE IN THE TREATMENT OF OBESITY FOR WEIGHT CONTROL. THERE IS NO SUBSTANTIAL EVIDENCE THAT HCG INCREASES WEIGHT LOSS BEYOND THAT RESULTING FROM CALORIC RESTRICTION, THAT IT CAUSES A MORE ATTRACTIVE OR "NORMAL" DISTRIBUTION OF FAT, OR THAT IT DECREASES THE HUNGER AND DISCOMFORT ASSOCIATED WITH CALORIE-RESTRICTIVE DIETS.

Since 1975, the FDA has required labeling and advertising of HCG to state: HCG has not been demonstrated to be an effective adjunctive therapy in the treatment of obesity. There is no substantial evidence that it increases weight loss beyond that resulting from caloric restriction, that it causes a more attractive or "normal" distribution of fat, or that it decreases the hunger and discomfort associated with calorie-restricted diets.

6. TERM: This license is effective from your date of purchase and shall remain in force until terminated. You may terminate the license and this License Agreement at any time by destroying the Licensed Product, together with all copies in any form. HCG Doctors Group, LLC may terminate this License Agreement if you breach any of the terms and conditions hereof. All provisions of this License Agreement relating to warranties, limitation of liability, proprietary rights and remedies or damages shall survive termination.

7. NO WAIVER. Any failure by either party to this License Agreement to enforce a specific part of the License Agreement in a specific situation is not a waiver of rights under this License Agreement. The party may still enforce the rest of the License Agreement in that situation and may still enforce some or all of the License Agreement in other situations.

8. This License Agreement constitutes the entire agreement between you and HCG Doctors Group, LLC pertaining to its subject matter. This License Agreement is governed by the laws of the State of Florida. Even if part of the License Agreement is held invalid, the rest of the License Agreement is still valid, binding and enforceable. LICENSEE ACKNOWLEDGES THAT LICENSEE HAS READ AND UNDERSTANDS THIS LICENSE AGREEMENT AND AGREES TO BE BOUND BY ITS TERMS. LICENSEE FURTHER AGREES THAT THIS LICENSE AGREEMENT IS THE COMPLETE AND EXCLUSIVE STATEMENT OF THE AGREEMENT BETWEEN LICENSEE AND I&P, AND SUPERSEDES ANY PROPOSAL OR PRIOR AGREEMENT, ORAL OR WRITTEN, AND ANY OTHER COMMUNICATIONS RELATING TO THE SUBJECT MATTER OF THIS AGREEMENT.

Medical Disclaimer: Although great care has been taken to provide informative material, be advised that any and all information and statements provided in this book is for informational purposes only and is not intended to diagnose, treat, cure or prevent any disease. The information presented is not intended to replace the advice provided by your own physician and in no way should be taken as Medical Advice.